Getting Preg

Improve Your Fertility
& Chances of IVF Success

Lois Francis.
Adv.Lic.Ac.,M.B.Ac.C.,P.G.C.E.,Cert.Counselling.,
Cert.N.L.P.,Cert.Nutrition

Why you should buy this book

Infertility is estimated to affect around one in six or one in seven couples in the UK – approximately 3.5 million people - at some point. Although the majority of these will become pregnant naturally given time, a significant minority will not.

Of 100 couples trying to conceive naturally:
20 will conceive within one month
70 will conceive within six months
85 will conceive within a year
90 will conceive within 18 months
95 will conceive within two years

Hi, I'm Lois Francis. I'm an acupuncturist with over 20 years experience of treating hundreds of patients who are struggling to get pregnant.   I've trained with renowned fertility expert Zita West and studied nutrition, in particular the work of Dr Marilyn Glenville and Patrick Holford.   I firmly believe that it's vital to take charge of your fertility by optimising your diet and lifestyle.

So many of my patients are given a diagnosis of "unexplained infertility", yet when we sit down together and go through their eating habits and lifestyle it becomes very obvious why they are struggling to get pregnant.

Time and again I've seen couples who have had failed fertility treatments in the past, improve their diets and go on to have a baby. Some have used assisted conception, but many find to their delight that they conceive naturally.

In this book I explain the diet and environmental factors that might be compromising your fertility and discuss what you can do to help yourself.

Many couples are simply unaware of the optimal time to try and conceive or how to monitor fertility signals. I explain this and how to chart your fertility.

I'll also de-mystify assisted conception and explain the various treatment options which are potentially available to you.

Free Guided Relaxations

One key thing I notice is the stress that couples are under when they are struggling to get pregnant. Stress is the enemy of fertility and so I always teach my patients ways to reduce their stress levels. In particular, when I am treating a woman through an IVF cycle I talk them through guided visualisation, according to where they are in the cycle.

Because my patients tell me that these relaxation sessions and guided visualisations are enormously helpful, I've included with this book twelve relaxation tracks which you can download from my website. Nine are for women, two for both of you and one for the men!

You'll find the download link in the resources section at the back of the book. I do hope you enjoy them and that they support you in your quest to become parents.

Lois Francis

The information in this book has the potential to improve not only your reproductive health, but also your general health. However, it should not be seen as a replacement for medical advice. If you have concerns about your health and fertility, please consult your medical practitioner.

ISBN: 9781549909481

PLANNING TO GET PREGNANT

In this first part of the book I'll explain the "mechanics" of fertility, the menstrual cycle and how to know when you are reaching peak fertile time.

We'll also look at testing for problems with your fertility and what all the test results mean to you.

UNDERSTANDING YOUR FERTILITY

For conception to take place you require a healthy egg, healthy sperm, intercourse at the fertile time in the woman's cycle and for an egg to be fertilised.

Conception occurs when the fertilised egg has embedded in the uterus. But what happens before then? Sperm can live for between 3 and 7 days whereas an egg is only capable of being fertilised for 8 to 12 hours. Timing of sex is crucial to your chances of getting pregnant. After ejaculation, the sperm begin the equivalent of a swimming marathon taking thousands of tail movements to move just 1 centimetre forward.

They are helped in their swim if sex has been timed to coincide with the woman's fertile secretions and they will take up to 2 hours to reach the egg in the fallopian tube. Sperm may rest at intervals and some may wait at the neck of the womb waiting for the egg to be released. At any one time there may be hundreds of sperm swimming round the egg, trying to "drill" their way in. Once a sperm has penetrated the egg, chemical changes mean that no other sperm can get in. The successful sperm sheds its protective head and the male and female cells merge.

From this point the fertilised egg continues on its way down the fallopian tube to embed in the uterus and so a new life begins.

THE ROLE OF REPRODUCTIVE HORMONES

For women there are 4 major hormones which control the phases of the menstrual cycle. These are Follicle Stimulating Hormone (FSH), Luteinising Hormone (LH), Oestrogen and Progesterone.

There are 3 phases in the cycle beginning with the Follicular phase which starts on day 1 of a woman's period. At the beginning of your menstrual cycle, whilst you have your period and up until ovulation, the hypothalamus produces gonadotropin-releasing hormone (GnRH).

The GnRH pulses through your bloodstream from the hypothalamus to the pituitary gland in spurts every 60-90 minutes from menstruation until ovulation. The GnRH signals the anterior pituitary gland to secrete Follicle Stimulating Hormone (FSH) and later Luteinizing Hormone (LH). You are generally not fertile at this time, the lining of the womb is shed to make ready for a fresh lining to build over the next few days.

The pituitary gland releases FSH and LH which stimulate the growth of about 15 to 20 eggs in the ovaries, each one contained within its own follicle. The follicular phase of your cycle extends from the beginning of the cycle until ovulation. FSH stimulates the development and maturation of follicles in the ovaries. One of these follicles will become dominant and contains the ovum that will be released at ovulation.

The oestrogen released by the developing follicles, and later by the dominant follicle, causes the lining of the uterus, the endometrium, to grow and thicken in preparation for implantation of a fertilized ovum.

By about the seventh day of your cycle on average (but this can vary widely) the dominant follicle takes over. The eggs within the other follicles lose their nourishment and die as do the follicular cells.

The dominant follicle produces a sharp rise in oestrogen. This usually coincides with changes in cervical fluid. Oestrogen is at its peak one to two days prior to ovulation.

The length of this phase can vary from woman to woman and from cycle to cycle. You are most fertile at the end of this phase during the days just before and including ovulation.

The ovulatory phase of the cycle begins when the surge in oestrogen signals the release of Luteinizing Hormone (LH). This is the hormone that is measured by ovulation predictor kits (OPKs). LH travels through the bloodstream to the ovary where it causes the ovary to release enzymes that make a hole in the sac of the dominant follicle.

This causes the dominant follicle to rupture and release the ovum into the fallopian tube where it can be fertilized. This is ovulation. The LH surge is necessary for ovulation to occur. The LH surge (the highest concentration of LH) occurs 12-24 hours prior to ovulation but LH begins to rise about 36 hours before ovulation.

As the egg travels down the fallopian tube it produces an enzyme that helps to attract and guide sperm toward it. Nature really tries to help us – this enzyme is almost like a homing device saying "here I am!"

Ovulation takes place, on average, about two weeks before your period, though it can vary from 10-16 days before the onset of menstruation depending on the length of your luteal phase. During an "average" 28 day cycle, ovulation is usually expected to take place between cycle days 13-15. Based on this guideline, we are taught to expect ovulation around day 14 of the menstrual cycle. Many women, however, do not have average cycles and even those who usually do, may see irregularities from time to time.

Once the egg is released, it is picked up by one of the fallopian tubes and begins to travel towards the uterus in the fallopian tube. This is where fertilization takes place. The follicle that released the egg becomes known as the corpus luteum after ovulation and begins to secrete the heat inducing hormone, progesterone to prepare the womb for a fertilised egg to implant.

Progesterone is the hormone that dominates this phase causing a rise in body temperature, which can be detected on your BBT chart. (There are now lots of Apps to help you plot your temperature and when you are likely to ovulate.)

Like oestrogen, progesterone is needed to develop the endometrium so that a fertilized egg can implant and be nourished should fertilization occur. Progesterone makes the lining of your uterus soft and spongy so that a fertilized egg can latch onto it and implant.

If an egg is fertilized and implantation of the fertilized egg occurs, the corpus luteum's life is extended. In conception cycles, the corpus luteum keeps on producing progesterone and some oestrogen and the development of the endometrium continues. The pregnancy hormone, hCG begins to be produced when the fertilized egg implants, at around 7-10 days after ovulation. As the pregnancy progresses, hormone production is taken over by the placenta.

Your BBT (Basal Body Temperature) rises as a result of progesterone production. If there is no pregnancy, the corpus luteum dies, progesterone levels fall, and a new cycle begins.

The luteal phase usually lasts 12-14 days but can last between 10-16 days. The length of this phase is fairly constant from cycle to cycle for the same woman. The length of the follicular phase may vary but the luteal phase length is generally constant. When cycles are irregular, it is usually because ovulation occurred earlier or later than usual.

You may have had your FSH levels checked already. High FSH levels (above 12) indicate that the ovaries are struggling and not responding to FSH.   More about tests later.

The primary hormones for a man are LH, FSH and testosterone.   FSH is needed to stimulate sperm production and a high FSH level can indicate that a man is struggling to make sperm. LH stimulates the production of testosterone, which in turn is responsible for male sexual development and arousal.

Understanding The Menstrual Cycle And Fertile Time

An average cycle is 28 days, but anything between 21 and 32 days is considered normal. The ideal period should be between 5 and 7 days with a flow of fresh, red blood and no clotting. The flow shouldn't be too light or too heavy and there shouldn't be significant pain or pre-menstrual tension. It's normal to have some breast or lower abdominal tenderness.

When you're trying to get pregnant, it's useful to keep a note of your periods. You want to know:

- if you have a regular cycle
- the length of your period
- the colour of the blood flow (red or brown etc)
- if you pass clots
- if you have significant pain with the period
- if you have mid-cycle pain or bleeding
- if you have any PMT – when do you get it and what symptoms do you experience?

According to American doctor, Dr Guy Abraham there are four main types of PMT:

Type A - Anxiety
This category is common in up to 80 per cent of women and includes symptoms such as mood swings, irritability, anxiety and tension. The effects

can be reduced to an extent by learning to use relaxation techniques. The guided relaxations that accompany the book can be a useful tool.

Type C - Cravings
This group includes cravings for sweets or chocolates, increased appetite, fatigue and headaches. Up to 60 per cent of women can experience these kinds of symptoms leading up to their period. It's important to keep blood sugar levels stable and following a low GL diet will help with this.

The recipes in the companion book "Eating to Get Pregnant" are all based on low GL.

Type H - Hyperhydration
Type H includes symptoms such as water retention, breast tenderness and enlargement, abdominal bloating and weight gain. Up to 40 per cent of women can experience these changes.

This can be related to high sodium and alcohol intake, so reducing salt and cutting back on the wine can help.

Type D - Depression
Depression is the largest symptom in this group but it can also include confusion, forgetfulness, clumsiness, withdrawal, lack of co-ordination, crying spells and confusion. Again, eating a low GL diet can help and avoiding stimulants such as caffeine and alcohol.

The herb Agnus Castus can improve PMT symptoms of irritability, mood alteration, anger, headache, and breast fullness by 50 per cent or more. It essentially raises progesterone levels and lowers oestrogen levels which are commonly out of balance and helps regulate the menstrual cycle.

Agnus castus also keeps prolactin secretion in check. The ability to decrease mildly elevated prolactin levels may benefit some infertile women as well as some women with breast tenderness associated with premenstrual syndrome (PMS).

Please note I would <u>always</u> recommend that you consult a qualified herbalist before taking any herb when you are trying to get pregnant.

In each menstrual cycle there is a "window of opportunity" in which you are most likely to conceive. This lasts about 5 to 6 days.

It seems that Nature plays a game with us, in that ovulation occurs <u>14 days before the start of your next period</u>. This is fine if your cycle is always regular, but can be tricky if you have irregular cycles.

Looking at an average 28 day cycle your window of opportunity looks something like this:-

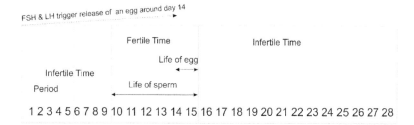

Under the influence of LH and FSH a follicle begins to ripen an egg. As the follicle produces more oestrogen, it causes FSH levels to drop and a surge in LH. The follicle ruptures and ovulation occurs. The ruptured follicle then produces progesterone until a fertilised egg has embedded in the uterus.

Once ovulation has occurred, the egg is caught by the fallopian tubes where it can survive for *up to 24 hours*, awaiting the arrival of sperm. On the other hand, sperm can survive *in the right alkaline cond*itions for up to 5 days.

The days when conception is possible are the days just before and including the day of ovulation. Based on the maximum lifespan of human sperm and ova, (five days for sperm and one day for the ovum) this fertile window is at MOST six days. This maximum window is made up of the five days before ovulation and the day of ovulation.

Though pregnancy is technically possible during this six day window, a more realistic fertile window is just 3 days. That is the 2 days before ovulation and the day of ovulation. Do remember that sperm will

10

survive, in optimum conditions for up to 5 days. Although you should focus on the 3 day window for intercourse, it's not the end of the world if you can only manage to have sex a few days earlier.

Begin to monitor the length of your cycle, so that you can determine when you are most likely to ovulate. If your cycle is 28 days, then you will most likely ovulate on day 14 counting from the first day of your period. If your cycle is 26 days you will ovulate on day 12 and if it is 32 days you will ovulate on day 18. You can see that the old idea of ovulating "mid-cycle" doesn't work for everyone!

You need to bear in mind that if you wait till you ovulate to have sex, then by the time the sperm complete their marathon swim, it may already be too late. In order to maximise your chances of getting pregnant, it is usually suggested that you have sex on alternate days in the lead up to ovulation.

THE IMPORTANCE OF REGULAR SEX

It's very easy when you are desperate to get pregnant to focus all your attention on having sex "at the right time." It's important to remember that you want a baby because you are in a supportive, loving relationship and that enjoying sex is part of that relationship.

Having sex regularly throughout your cycle helps to keep stress under control, and makes sure that in your fertile time you have sperm which are fresh and vigourous.

Make love every second day from the end of your period and up to 5 or 6 days post ovulation. Love making and intimacy help you produce oxytocin.

Often referred to as the "love molecule", oxytocin is typically associated with helping couples establish a greater sense of intimacy and attachment. Oxytocin, along with dopamine and norepinephrine, are believed to be highly critical in human pair-bonding.

But not only that, it also increases the desire for couples to gaze at one another, it creates sexual arousal, and it helps males maintain their erections. When you're sexually aroused or excited, oxytocin levels increase in your brain significantly — a primary factor for bringing about an orgasm. And during the orgasm itself, the brain is flooded with oxytocin — a possible explanation for why couples like to cuddle after.

Critically, oxytocin is known to reduce stress hormones, which is hugely beneficial when you're focussed on trying to get pregnant. Remember that cuddles, caresses, kisses and general closeness to each other will help you both produce oxytocin.

Don't worry about making love "too often".

Remember that men make sperm 24/7 at the rate of approximately 50,000 a minute, so although each ejaculate contains up to 300 million sperm there are plenty more being made! If a man does not ejaculate for 4 to 5 days or longer, the sperm get caught in a "backlog" and their quality deteriorates. It can then take 2 ejaculations to "clear the tubes".

Making love every 48 hours will give time for the sperm count to top up to full capacity. It's also important for the health of the prostate gland that a man has regular ejaculations.

Healthy vigorous sperm swim at a speed of 2 to 3mm per minute and usually reach the fallopian tube within 2 hours. Seminal fluid contains nutrients which can help sperm stay alive for up to 6 or 7 days waiting for the egg to be released.   Having sex on alternate days during your "window of opportunity" will maximise your chances of getting pregnant.   The more sperm there are available, the more likely you are to catch the egg whilst it is capable of being fertilised.

Frequent sex does not weaken sperm. The chances of conception per cycle increase from around 15% for couples having sex once a week to around 50% for couples having sex every day, (lower % for older couples). Sperm quality deteriorates if they are retained in a man's tubes for more than about 3 days, so frequent ejaculation through the cycle ensures that there are fresh healthy sperm available at the fertile time.

Enjoying sex and achieving orgasm can help conception. This may be due to the effect of the contractions during orgasm helping to 'suck up' the sperm. Many women find it easier to relax and have an orgasm when they are less stressed, such as on holiday. So if possible try to keep sex spontaneous, varied, passionate and fun.

Stay flat after intercourse: When the seminal fluid is ejaculated it is a viscous consistency. This sticks to the woman's cervix, but then within a few moments, it liquefies releasing the sperm. The strong healthy sperm start to swim rapidly through the fertile secretions in the woman's cervix.

The rest of the seminal fluid and the weaker and dying sperm will leak back out of the vagina about 10-15 minutes after intercourse. There is no evidence that pillows under buttocks or any other gymnastic feats will help, but it makes sense to stay flat for about 15 minutes. Avoid leaping straight out of bed, wiping or washing immediately.

Recognising Your Fertility Signals

There is one very straightforward way to recognise when you are entering your fertile window of opportunity. The mucus secreting glands which line your cervix produce mucus continuously and they are part of the self-cleansing mechanism of the vagina.

During the follicular phase of the menstrual cycle the mucus is thick and sticky forming a plug over the cervix which prevents sperm from entering. It also makes the vagina more acid which kills off sperm.

This is a perfect time to have fun sex, staying connected with each other and making sure that you have fresh virile sperm when you reach peak fertile time.

When the sticky plug comes away from the cervix it indicates that the fertile time is starting. Cervical secretions increase by a factor of 10. At first they feel moist or sticky and look white or cloudy. As they become clearer, wetter, slippery and stretchy you are in your most fertile time. After ovulation the secretions revert to sticky, then dry.

It can help to wear black or red knickers so you can see the mucus more clearly. As the cervical secretions get wetter, the PH level in the vagina begins to change, making it more sperm friendly.

The fertile secretions turn the vaginal fluids alkaline and provide nourishment for sperm in the form of sugar, amino acids, salt and water enabling them to live for up to 7 days.   Fertile mucus also contains "swimming lanes" through which sperm can travel easily.   At this time the cervix is lifting making the journey for the sperm shorter.

Fertile mucus is a pre-cursor to ovulation and is produced around 12 to 48 hours before an egg is released.

To identify fertile mucus, use white toilet paper to blot your vaginal mucus after passing urine.   If it feels slippery like raw egg white and can stretch between your fingers, it is fertile mucus.   If it is dry, thick, sticky, crumbly, opaque, white or yellow in colour is is the more acid, infertile mucus.

There are many factors that can have an impact on your production of cervical mucus:

- Anti-histamine or diuretic medication (because they are drying up secretions generally)
- The fertility drug Clomid (Clomiphene)
- Tamoxifen
- GnRH agonists
- Progesterones
- Tranquillisers
- Anti-biotics
- Expectorants in cough medicines

- Vitamin C in excess of 1000mg a day as it has an anti-histamine effect and can make cervical secretions more acidic
- Use of tampons and panty liners
- G string panties
- Vaginal or sexually transmitted infections
- Vaginal douching
- Being overweight
- Breastfeeding (high prolactin levels can suppress oestrogen secretion)
- Decreased ovarian function

The day after having sex you may notice some white or clear discharge which is liquefied semen, but can easily be confused with cervical mucus, as can vaginal secretions produced when you are sexually aroused. If you're not sure if you have fertile secretions, put some in a glass of water - they will stay in a blob if they are cervical secretions, otherwise they will dissolve.

Doing pelvic floor exercises can help you detect changes in your mucus. Tighten the pelvic floor muscles, hold for a few seconds and then relax. In the most fertile time you will notice a slippery feel between your legs as you do this exercise.

If you're not sure which are your pelvic floor muscles, imagine that you need to go to the toilet urgently for a wee, but there is no toilet facility available. It's the muscles you use to hold your wee that are your pelvic floor muscles.

Make a habit of exercising these muscles every day as they can be challenged during childbirth, sneezing, coughing or jumping up and down. Toned pelvic floor muscles can also intensify sexual pleasure. (By the way, if you belong to a gym that has a power plate, you can sit on the power plate and get some good exercising of your pelvic floor muscles.)

Whilst we are talking about cervical secretions, it's worth mentioning that most proprietary vaginal lubricants are hostile to sperm. Saliva (yours or his) contains digestive enzymes and can kill off sperm. Tap water, baby oil, mineral oil or egg white can also damage sperm.

If you need to use some lubrication, look for one that specifically says it is fertility friendly. Pre-Seed is designed for use by couples trying to conceive and is available from Amazon both in America and the UK.

To maximise your production of cervical mucus, make sure that you drink plenty of water, at least 1½ litres a day, and that you have at least 5 portions of fruit and vegetables daily. Avoid acid foods such as sugar, caffeine and cola drinks. Evening Primrose Oil can be taken from day 1 of your period up to ovulation to help with the production of cervical mucus. You can take 1500 to 3000mg daily, provided that you have not been diagnosed with high oestrogen levels.

Don't worry if you can't detect your cervical secretions, monitor the length of your cycle, get a clear idea of your window of opportunity and aim to have sex every other day at that time.

SECONDARY FERTILITY SIGNS

The most frequently noted additional signs are:

Ovulation Pain: Not everyone feels ovulation pain. It may be felt as a slight pain that you feel near your abdomen or ovary around the time of ovulation. It does not necessarily occur at the exact time of ovulation but may happen up to a few days before, during or soon after ovulation. Because of this, ovulation pain is useful only to cross-check other signs, but cannot be used to definitively confirm or pinpoint ovulation.

Increased Sex Drive: If you notice that there is a pattern to your sex drive, it can be helpful to record your observations to make predictions about your fertility. Some women notice that their sex drive is highest at around the time when they are most fertile.

Ovulation spotting: Some women see slight spotting at the time of ovulation. This is quite rare, but you may see that your cervical fluid is streaked with blood or has a pink tinge. If you do notice this, it should be noted. If it is heavy, unusual for you, or lasts longer than a day or is otherwise a cause for concern, you should ask your doctor about it.

Tender Breasts: The sensitivity of your breasts may be useful for you to cross-check other signs if you have a consistent pattern but it is not a useful fertility sign on its own. You may notice that your breasts feel more sensitive at around the time of ovulation and they may continue to feel sensitive or tender throughout your luteal phase.

If you notice that there is an observable pattern to the sensitivity of your breasts, it is useful to record it so that you can make future predictions or notice changes from cycle to cycle. For some women, tender breasts are an early pregnancy symptom, however, there is no way to know if you are pregnant by the sensitivity of your breasts.

Breast sensitivity may be linked to increased progesterone. Progesterone is increased both during the luteal phase of your menstrual cycle when you are not pregnant and during pregnancy.

Your own observations: You may notice some specific changes yourself that can offer clues about your fertility pattern. Everyone is different, but there are clues that you may find on your own. Changes in your complexion, your energy level, your moods, or anything else that you notice shows a cyclical pattern can offer insight into your fertility pattern. Record any such observations on your chart. You may be surprised to learn that something seemingly unrelated may be related to your fertility.

TEMPERATURE CHARTS

These can be useful to help monitor when ovulation is occurring and that your progesterone levels are rising in the luteal phase of your cycle. You should take your temperature <u>at the same time every morning</u> before you get out of bed.

Your temperature is lowest around 3 to 4am and rises .1 degree every hour after that. Having a late meal, alcohol, illness, stress, anxiety, fever, shift working, paracaetamol, aspirin, getting up in the night can all affect the temperature reading. You must be in bed at least 3 hours before you take your temperature to get accurate readings.

Temperature rises between 0.5 and 1 degree after ovulation and there is often a slight dip just before ovulation. The rise in temperature is due to the influence of progesterone which is trying to make the womb warm and receptive to a fertilised egg.

I usually suggest to my patients that they consider charting for around 3 months to get familiar with their unique cycle and fertility signals. The more aware you become of your fertile window, the easier it is to time intercourse to make the most of your chances of conceiving.

I only suggest charting for 3 months if your pattern is pretty stable from month to month. Then put the charts away, keep a mental note of when your next fertile window will be and get on with enjoying life!

The resources section at the back of the book gives you a full explanation of how to chart and monitor your temperature.

OVULATION TEST KITS

Luteinizing Hormone (LH) is the last hormone to peak before ovulation and is the hormone responsible for triggering the rupture of the ovarian sac that releases the egg at ovulation. This hormone can be measured by ovulation prediction kits (OPKs) and fertility monitors that use chemicals to identify its presence in your urine.

The presence of increased amounts of LH in your urine, as detected by OPKs, usually means that you will ovulate within 12-24 hours but this can vary slightly depending on your own hormonal profile. LH is not released all at once, but rather it rises and falls for about 24-48 hours.

The LH rise usually begins in the early morning while you are sleeping and it takes 4-6 hours for it to appear in your urine after that. For this reason, first morning urine may not give the best result. Testing mid-day is usually recommended. It is important to follow the instructions of your OPK for maximum results.

Many women like ovulation prediction kits, even though they are not able to confirm or pinpoint ovulation precisely, because they can tell you that ovulation is imminent.

It is important, however, not to rely exclusively on OPKs for timing intercourse and identifying your most fertile time. This is because you may already be fertile before your OPK turns positive. You may like to use them to cross-check your other fertility signs and to offer additional clues about impending ovulation.

They may be especially useful if you have ambiguous charts. If your cycles are irregular or very long, OPKs may be very costly because you may need to use several tests to be sure to catch the LH surge.

Following a few guidelines can help you get the most out of your OPK:

Like any product, follow the manufacturer's instructions carefully.

If you do not test every day from before you expect to be most fertile, you may miss the surge. Likewise, if you test too late, you may miss the surge.

Testing daily once you have started to test is the best strategy. Your first positive OPK result probably means that you are about to ovulate. Since OPK packages include only a limited number of test strips and are fairly expensive, timing when to start testing is crucial.

Follow the manufacturer's instructions about the time to take your OPK. First morning urine is usually not the best for OPKs since your LH surge usually begins in early morning when you are still sleeping and may not be apparent in your first morning urine. If you test in the early morning, you may miss your surge entirely since LH levels may already be reduced by the next morning. Late morning or early afternoon is usually best unless the instructions (or your doctor) suggest otherwise.

Unless the manufacturer's instructions suggest otherwise, record your OPK results as positive if the test line is as dark as or darker than the control line. Record your results as negative if the test line is lighter than the control line. For digital tests, follow the manufacturer's directions.

Do not rely exclusively on OPK results to time intercourse as you may not see an LH surge (positive OPK) even though you may be fertile. Your increased fertility begins before you see a positive OPK result since sperm can live in the reproductive tract for a few days in fertile cervical fluid.

Ovulation kits only identify a short time from the surge in LH to ovulation.   Waiting till you get the "go ahead" from an ovulation kit can mean that you have let most of your fertile window pass by and so missed an opportunity. Remember that the egg is only available to be fertilised for a matter of hours, and that you need to get sperm "in situ" well ahead of time!

During your potentially fertile time, have intercourse at least every other day even before you see a positive OPK result. Switch to every single day once you see a positive result until ovulation has been confirmed by your temperature data. (Talk to your doctor about intercourse frequency if you suspect any sperm issues).

If you are taking Clomid, ask your doctor or the OPK manufacturer when to start testing with OPKs.

Don't even consider saliva testing devices – a study published in the Lancet found that 8/10 post menopausal women and 10/10 men tested positive for ovulation!

One old fashioned method (pre-ovulation test kits) was to use litmus paper to test the acidity/alkalinity of the vagina. It should change to being more alkaline as the cervical secretions increase. Again, it can be a way to help identify the fertile window, but don't get hooked on using it.

Your doctor can do blood tests to check that you are ovulating. These are usually done mid-way through the second half of your cycle (around day 21). Another test is usually done to check your follicle stimulating hormone (FSH) level and other hormones and blood levels on days 1-3 of your cycle. The timing of these tests is crucial. Women with irregular cycles may have problems timing the tests accurately.

Acupuncture can help to boost natural fertility by balancing hormones, improving blood flow to the reproductive organs and boosting egg growth and the thickness of the womb lining. It can also help to improve the quality of sperm. It's really good for reducing stress too.

UNDERSTANDING MALE FERTILITY

In the past, many fertility clinics tended to focus on problems with the female partner, yet problems with male fertility account for between 30 and 35% of cases.

I believe that if you are to create a healthy baby, then both partners need to optimise their fertility and the health of the eggs and sperm. It can come as quite a shock (and blow to the ego) for a man to find that a sperm analysis reveals problems with his fertility.

Unlike women who are born with their egg reserve, men do not begin to produce sperm until puberty (usually around age 12 to 14). When puberty is reached the pituitary gland produces follicle stimulating hormone (FSH) and luteinizing hormone

(LH). It is these 2 hormones that stimulate the ovaries in a woman and the testes in a man.

FSH and LH stimulate the testes to produce sperm and testosterone which is responsible for the development of adult male characteristics such as facial and body hair, and a deepening of the voice. Testosterone influences the strengthening of muscles, emotions and of course sex drive.

However, high testosterone levels and a high sex drive don't necessarily equate to high fertility or good sperm quality.

In all it takes around 100 days for the sperm production process. 74 days for the sperm to develop and a further 20 to 30 days for them to reach maturity. Men are continually producing sperm, so there is much that can be done to improve their quality.

In the 74 day development period the sperm grow a head which contains the DNA and the X or Y chromosome which determines the sex of the baby. The middle piece contains their energy source which feeds the long tail used for propulsion.

The seminal glands and prostate produce fluids, which when combined with the sperm is referred to as semen. The fluid produced by the prostate gland is slightly alkaline, helping to counteract the acid secretions of the woman's vagina and thus protect the sperm.

The seminal fluid contains nutrients to help nourish and feed the sperm as they make their way toward the egg. Around 250 million sperm are released with each ejaculation, of these only about 1 million reach the cervix and around 200 reach the fallopian tube and the egg. It really is survival of the fittest!

I sometimes wonder if nature deliberately made the journey to the egg so hard in order to ensure that only the best sperm could reach the egg and fertilise it!

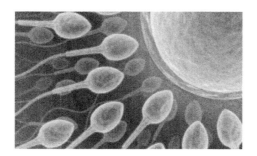

CHECKING FOR PROBLEMS WITH YOUR FERTILITY

Sadly, problems with fertility have significantly increased over the past few years, with as many as 25% of couples experiencing difficulty conceiving.

The diagnosis of "unexplained infertility" now accounts for a massive 30% of the diagnoses made by the medical profession. This is closely followed by problems with the man's fertility, ovulation problems, fallopian tube damage and endometriosis.

According to the HFEA statistics, the reasons for infertility are:

Male factor – 40%

Female factor – 40%

Multiple male and female factors – 10.8%

Unexplained infertility – 30%

Other factors – 1.1%

Some couples may have a combination of factors affecting their chances of conception. If you've been given a diagnosis of unexplained infertility, you may be relieved to know that there is a lot you can do to improve both partners fertility. This diagnosis can be viewed as a golden opportunity to take a serious look at your general and reproductive health and make positive changes.

If you are under 35 and you've been trying for a year to conceive, then you may be referred for tests. If you are over 35 and have been trying for 6 months, then you should visit your GP sooner to ask for tests.

There is a battery of tests for women to check for infections, ovulation, blocked tubes etc. and for men the semen analysis. Both partners should be tested at the same time.

FACTORS WHICH MAY AFFECT FEMALE FERTILITY AND RECURRENT MISCARRIAGE.

- Hormone imbalances due to nutritional deficiencies

- Anaemia

- Coeliac disease

- Diabetes

- Endometriosis

- Polycystic ovaries

- Fibroids, cysts, polyps

- Immune system disorders

- Recurrent miscarriage

- Smoking

- Alcohol

- Drug use

- BMI too low or too high

- Genetic disease

- Serious illness

- Blood clotting disorders

- STIs or GUIs

- Exposure to X-ray

- Long periods in aeroplanes

- Exposure to toxins and chemicals. This can be work related – workers in chemical factories, hairdressers etc.

- Overuse of laxatives

THE COMMON FEMALE TESTS.

FSH – Your FSH level will be checked by a blood test, usually around day 2 or 3 of your cycle. Ideally, your FSH level should be below 10. In general a reading of:

Under 6 is excellent

6 – 9 is good

 9 – 10 is fair

10 – 13 diminished reserve

13+ very hard to stimulate.

Anything higher than that indicates that your ovaries are not responding well to FSH and that your pituitary gland is producing more to try and stimulate development of a follicle.

Fertility clinics in general like the FSH level to be no higher than 10 as this could be a predictor of poor response to fertility drugs. However, a higher FSH level does **not** mean that you can't get pregnant, even with an FSH level of 12 to 14 you can still get pregnant.

Following the guidance in this book there is much you can do to improve both your FSH level and the quality of the eggs you produce.

If your FSH level is high it may be a sign of:

Premature menopause

Poor ovarian reserve

LH – Luteinising hormone (LH) is the hormone that is released to trigger ovulation and is the hormone that is measured with ovulation test kits. It's usually tested on days 1 to 5 of your cycle. High levels of LH may suggest PCOS.

Prolactin – this hormone is released by the pituitary gland to prepare the breasts for milk production. It is usually present in high levels when a woman is breast feeding and it suppresses ovulation, which is why many women do not have periods when breast feeding.

If high prolactin levels are found this can be an indication of an underactive thyroid. Stress can be a factor as high levels of stress hormones can cause a reduction in the secretion of dopamine which in turn can raise prolactin levels. Low levels of dopamine can also cause a loss of libido.

Oestradiol – This hormone is a form of oestrogen and it causes the lining of the womb to thicken in readiness for implantation. It's usually measured on day 1 to 3 and ideally should be low. When the oestradiol reading is below 180 pmol/L this will give a true reading for FSH.

Thyroid hormones – if your thyroid is underactive this can lead to heavy, longer periods or a shorter cycle. If it's severe it can stop ovulation, periods or cause irregular periods. TSH levels should be less than 2 for optimum fertility. If it is over 2, you can consider taking kelp tablets.

Thyroid function is important for controlling all the metabolic processes in the body. A borderline underactive thyroid may show increased TSH levels with normal T4 levels. A good diet is essential for normal thyroid function, making sure to include foods rich in B vitamins and the minerals magnesium, chromium, selenium, zinc and calcium.

Common symptoms of underactive thyroid are:

- Fatigue

- Weakness

- Weight gain or difficulty losing weight

- Coarse dry hair

- Dry, rough pale skin

- Hair loss

- Intolerance to cold

- Muscle cramps and aches

- Constipation

- Depression

- Irritability

- Memory loss

- Abnormal menstrual cycles

- Decreased libido

If you have 2 or more of these symptoms, it is worth getting your thyroid hormones checked.

Progesterone – At day 21 of your cycle (assuming you have a 28 day cycle) your progesterone levels are checked by blood test to make sure that you are ovulating. A level of 30 or more suggests that you are ovulating. A level below 5 indicates that no ovulation has occurred.

Infections – both partners should be screened for a range of infections which can affect your fertility. These include Chlamydia, bacterial infections, streptococci, toxoplasmosis, STDs. You should also be checked for immunity to German measles.

HyCoSy – a vaginal ultrasound scan in which a small catheter is passed through the cervix into the uterus. Fluid is passed through the catheter into the fallopian tubes and an ultrasound scan can pick up if there are any blockages. This test is usually carried out in the first half of your cycle when you can be sure that you are not already pregnant.

AMH – Anti-mullerian hormone or AMH is made by the ovaries to help eggs mature each month. It also plays a role in the production of oestrogen. The AMH test is a good indicator of how well your ovaries are functioning, the quantity and quality of your egg reserves.

AMH levels do not change significantly throughout the menstrual cycle and decrease with age. Healthy women, below 38 years old, with normal follicular status at day 3 of the menstrual cycle, have AMH levels of 2.0 - 6.8 ng/ml (14.28 - 48.55 pmol/L). High levels are found in patients with PCOS. The lower the level of AMH the lower your fertility is likely to be.

Interpretation	AMH ng/ml	AMH pmol/L
Optimal fertility	4 – 6.8	28.6 – 48.5
Satisfactory fertility	2.2 - 4	15.7 – 28.6
Low fertility	0.3 – 2.2	2.2 – 15.7
Very low/undetectable	0 – 0.3	0.0 – 2.2
High level	➢ 6.8	➢ 48.5 pmol/L

Do bear in mind that a low AMH level is only an *indicator*. There is much you can do to improve the quality of your eggs if you follow the advice in this book.

You may also be offered scans to check that you are ovulating and that the corpus luteum, which produces progesterone after release of the egg, is functioning normally. Usually, if these tests are negative, i.e. no problem has been found, you may be offered I.U.I. or IVF treatment.

PCOS AND ENDOMETRIOSIS

Polycystic Ovarian Syndrome (PCOS) is a condition where multiple cysts cover the ovaries that are filled with immature follicles (eggs). It is associated with hormonal abnormalities and irregularities in ovulation and menstruation. It is a metabolic condition associated with insulin resistance and glucose intolerance.

Common symptoms of PCOS are:

- failure to ovulate

- acne

- obesity or difficulty maintaining correct weight

- irregular periods

- excessive facial or body hair

If PCOS is severe, you may have all of the symptoms while mild and moderate cases only have some.

PCOS can cause infertility because there are too many male hormones (androgens, testosterone) and not enough oestrogen and progesterone, so follicles don't mature and ovulate.

Insulin resistance has been found to contribute to excess production of androgens by the ovaries. Insulin resistance goes hand in hand with obesity or being overweight especially around the middle (visceral fat = fat around the organs). However insulin resistance can also be found among people who are not obese or overweight. If you are overweight and have PCOS infertility it is advisable that that you lose weight and correct insulin resistance.

Insulin resistance means that the cells are not responding to insulin when it tries to remove excess glucose from the bloodstream and deposit it into the cells. A diet that is high in refined and simple carbohydrates is usually the source of the problem.

When the cells fail to respond to insulin and take in the glucose, it leads to excess glucose in the blood stream and not enough in the cells. This in turn leads to fatigue and lethargy and increased risk of diabetes.

Too much glucose in the bloodstream is potentially very damaging to your organs.

If you have too much LH and not enough FSH being produced, it leads to immature eggs which never reach the ovulation stage and end up forming small cysts on the ovaries. It will also cause an excess of testosterone.

Normalizing your hormones and getting your body to produce sufficient amount of hormones to ovulate and maintain pregnancy is the key to treating PCOS infertility.

Studies have found that the majority of cases of infertility due to ovulatory disorders may be prevented with dietary and lifestyle modifications. The guidance in this book and the companion book Eating to Get Pregnant will help to regulate your insulin levels.

The general diet and lifestyle principles are:

- Every 3 hours to balance your blood sugar

- Eat Small Protein Rich Meals

- Exercise Regularly doing cardio and weights (the more muscles you have the more fat you'll burn).

- Minimise your intake of dairy and animal products

Endometriosis

Endometriosis is a painful condition which can impact fertility. Endometrial cells from the lining of the uterus migrate to other areas in the pelvic cavity where they don't belong. Endometriosis is one of the most frequent diseases in gynaecology, affecting 15-20% of women in their reproductive life, contributing to 5% cases of infertility.

Endometrial tissue growth is usually found in the lower abdomen, it can attach to the ovaries, ligaments, fallopian tubes, bowel and bladder. It has even been found in the lungs, though this is uncommon.

Wherever the endometrial tissue is in the body, it responds to hormone signals and bleeds during menstruation. This blood is unable to leave the body in the way that menstrual blood normally would and so it forms scar tissue and adhesions.

Endometriosis can cause heavy and painful periods, abnormal bleeding and infertility.

There are a few theories as to how the tissue manages to migrate. Some suggesting retrograde flow of menstrual blood and seeding or attaching to other tissues, while others suggest endometrial cells being laid down in the wrong places during the embryologic development of the fetus. This theory emerged as it could not be explained how endometrial tissue reached the brain though the retrograde flow of menstrual blood.

Many women experience retrograde flow into the abdominal cavity via the fallopian tubes, but this is usually "mopped up" by the immune system. Yet another theory suggests that endometrial growths start from stem cells and are caused by a combination of factors.

As endometriosis has been associated with the presence of auto-antibodies and the presence of other autoimmune diseases, scientists are now suggesting that endometriosis is an autoimmune disease.

Although genetic predisposition, environmental factors and altered immune and endocrine function are believed to play a significant role in endometriosis, the true cause still remains unclear.

If the endometrial tissue grows within the fallopian tubes it can block them. Due to inflammation there are a high number of macrophages (the immune system "mopping up" cells) in the area which can destroy the sperm and interfere with implantation.

Ovulation may or may not occur, and even if it does occur there may not be enough progesterone to support the implantation. The risk of ectopic pregnancy is higher than usual. Anti-endometrial antibodies may be responsible for the high incidence of miscarriages and poor implantation often associated with this condition.

Five Tips For Getting Pregnant With Endometriosis

The natural treatment of endometriosis incorporates diet, detoxification, supplementation and exercise. Endometriosis is viewed as an oestrogen dependent condition and the endometrial implants have been shown to reduce in size when oestrogen levels in the body normalize or drop. Studies have found that inflammation resulting from bleeding of the endometrial implants each month actually increases oestrogen activity. Another contributing factor is low progesterone which can lead to anovulatory cycles.

1. Eat organically grown food and avoid exposure to commercial insect repellants.

2. Avoid soft plastics.

3. Reduce your intake of animal products.

4. Support your immune system by taking supplements which contain vitamin C, vitamin E, betacarotene, zinc and selenium and probiotics.

5. Take a high quality fish oil (make sure the one you choose is tested for mercury and stabilized with vitamin E (to protect it from oxidation). Fish oil reduces inflammation associated with endometriosis, minimizing associated pain and improving the odds of healthy implantation.

Factors Which May Affect Male Fertility

Varioceles. These are enlarged veins around the testes which can inhibit sperm production and possibly their motility.

Damage to the testes

Genetic or birth defects

STIs or GUIs

Mumps before or during puberty

Retrograde ejaculation due to damaged nerves, diabetes, STIs.

Impotence or inability to ejaculate.

Male Tests. - Semen Analysis

Male sperm count is dropping world wide. In 1935 the count was 135 million per ml. 20 years ago it fell to 30 million per ml. and is now 20 million per ml.

If the sperm count is below 20 million you may be considered sub-fertile. It is below 13.5 million you may be considered infertile.

At the end of 2009 the World Health Organization (WHO) published new reference guidelines for semen parameters. These guidelines were generated by evaluating 4,500 men in 14 countries whose partners had less than or equal to 12 months time to pregnancy (TTP). WHO found that with a 95% confidence, men whose partners had TTP of 12 or fewer months had NO LESS than the following:

Semen volume: 1.5 ml

Total sperm in the ejaculate: 39 million

Sperm per ml: 15 million/ml

Vitality: 58% live

Progressive motility: 32%

Total Motility: 40%

Morphologically Normal: 4%

If you have been trying to conceive for a while (at least 6 months) it is important that you are both investigated. Male infertility is the sole cause of failing to conceive in as much as 35% of cases and a contributory factor in 30 - 40% of cases. You should refrain from ejaculating for 2 days before giving your sample for analysis.

An analysis will give you sperm count, motility and morphology. It will also assess your seminal volume, the PH, white blood cells, round cells, agglutination of sperm, antisperm antibodies, debris, liquefaction and viscosity of the sample.

Ideally, you are looking for:

Semen volume: around 2ml

Sperm per ml: over 20 million

Total Motility: (how many of them are actually moving) should be more than 50%, with at least 25% having rapid progression.

Morphologically Normal: At least 15% should be of normal shape.

Volume

The normal volume is 2ml or about half a teaspoon. If the volume is too low, this can affect the transportation of the sperm and they may not reach the egg. If the volume is too high, this causes a dilution in the concentration of sperm and can affect their motion.

Sperm Count

The average count per ml is 60 – 80 million, but a count of 20 million is considered to be adequate for a woman to get pregnant.

Motility

This is a measure of how well the sperm are moving, that they move quickly and in a straight line. Motility of the sperm can be affected by lifestyle factors such as drinking alcohol. A long period without ejaculating will result in a higher percentage of dead or immobile sperm in the semen sample.

Sperm motility is classified as follows:-

A) Rapid progression where healthy sperm move at a good speed and in a straight line.

B) There is movement but it is slow or erratic.

C) The sperm show slight twitchy movements but do not move forward.

D) No movement of the sperm.

Ideally you want at least 50% of the sperm in category A or B and at least 25% in category A.

Morphology (Shape)

The sperm morphology relates to the number of normal/abnormal sperm, the number of normal sperm should be greater than 15%. Abnormal sperm can have malformations in the tail where it can be coiled, thickened or a double tail, disabling the sperm. (This is more common in older men.)

The head of the sperm which carries the genetic material should be oval, the midpiece normal and the tail long. A round, pin, large or double head may make fertilisation impossible.

The morphology of the sperm is often considered to be more important than the quantity. Many problems are due to lifestyle and diet factors, excessive exercise and excessive heat.

Following the advice in this booklet can significantly improve sperm count, motility and morphology.

MAR test

Stands for Mixed Antiglobulin Reaction. Fewer than 10% of spermatozoa should have adherent particles of antibodies. Antibodies in blood, semen or cervical mucus coat the surface of the sperm, which impairs swimming and the ability of the sperm to penetrate the egg.

If the man has had any trauma, surgery or infection in the groin area antibodies to the sperm may be produced. This can cause agglutination (sperm sticking together), decrease sperm motility and affect fertilization.

If 50% or more of the mobile sperm have antibodies attached to them, this may be diagnosed as immunological infertility. Steroids may help lower antibody levels but assisted conception may be needed. Most clinics wash and separate sperm to remove those with antibodies, so they may not offer this test to you.

If the woman has high levels of antibodies in her cervical mucus, she may be given steroid treatment.

The semen analysis will also check the ph of the semen which should be alkaline; agglutination i.e. if the sperm are clumping or sticking together; antisperm antibodies; how quickly the semen becomes liquid and the viscosity i.e. thickness of the semen.

DIETARY, LIFESTYLE & ENVIRONMENTAL FACTORS THAT AFFECT FERTILITY

I can't emphasis enough the importance of getting your diet right, not just during pregnancy, but in the pre-conception period when sperm and eggs are developing.

Poor nutrition in pregnancy and in the pre-conception period programmes the unborn child for health problems in later life.

An international study, led by Professor Keith Godfrey of University of Southampton showed that a mother's diet can alter the function of her child's DNA. The process, called epigenetic change, can lead to her child tending to lay down more fat. Importantly, the study showed that this effect acts *independently of how fat or thin the mother is* and of the child's weight at birth.

The epigenetic changes, which alter the *function* of our DNA without changing the actual DNA sequence inherited from the mother and father, can also influence how a person responds to lifestyle factors such as diet or exercise and their risk of developing diseases in adult life.

So what does this mean? The study was clear that the weight of the mother was not an influencing factor, rather it was the *quality* of her diet. The food she put into her mouth became her eggs, her developing baby. The way that the child's DNA functions and therefore his/her health is a direct result of what she ate both before and during pregnancy.

Clearly, what you put in your mouth is important. But of equal importance are the toxic foods which you **must** leave out if you are to achieve your dream of getting pregnant **and** have a healthy child.

THE TOXIC "FOODS" AND DRINKS

Aspartame and all artificial sweeteners should be eliminated from your diet. Sorry, but artificial sweeteners are just as bad as sugar. They all break down into deadly acids in your body.

One of the most common sweeteners is aspartame. One of its ingredients, methyl alcohol, converts into formaldehyde which is a deadly neurotoxin and known carcinogen. (And yes, you're right formaldehyde is used to embalm dead bodies.)

Formaldehyde turns into formic acid which is the poison that fire ants use! Hmmm, do you begin to wonder what place aspartame has in our food and drinks?

Artificial sweeteners have been shown to cause a wide array of symptoms such as:

- Headaches

- migraines
- dizziness
- vertigo
- seizures
- depression
- fatigue
- palpitations
- irritability
- insomnia
- vision problems
- <u>weight gain</u>
- joint pain
- anxiety attacks

to name just a few!

Artificial sweeteners can also trigger or worsen arthritis, chronic fatigue syndrome, diabetes, fibromyalgia, brain tumours, MS, Parkinson's disease, Alzheimer's disease, systemic lupus, mental retardation, **birth defects**, thyroid disorders and epilepsy.

It is thought to accumulate in the cells, *causing damage to the cell DNA.*

Sadly, many people use artificial sweeteners in the (mistaken) belief that it will help them lose weight. Your body simply doesn't understand chemicals in food or drink. So if something tastes sweet, it assumes that that "something" is sugar and that there is too much sugar in the bloodstream. Your pancreas releases insulin to take the "excess sugar" out of the blood and dump it into fat stores, leaving you feeling hungry.

Formaldehyde preserves fat cells in the body making it impossible for the body to break them down. So not only do people who use aspartame not lose weight, it keeps you constantly hungry and also preserves the fat you already have! Aspartame is the most controversial food additive in history, the American FDA refused approval 8 times before succumbing to industry pressure.

Sugar and sweeteners can get hidden in the most unlikely places and so you have to be vigilant and check EVERYTHING that you buy. I've even found aspartame in multivitamin supplements! Used in over 5,000 products, most commonly you'll find them in soft drinks, pop, soda, sauces (both sweet and savoury), cream, ice cream, cereal products, biscuits, cookies, cakes, candy bars and, wait for it, weightwatchers products! Generally any 'sugar-free' product or 'without added sugar' will contain an artificial sweetener.

MSG (monosodium glutamate) is used as a flavour enhancer in a wide range of products. It can be found in:

- soy sauce
- sauces

- gravies
- low-fat and no-fat milk
- candy
- gum
- processed food
- flavoured noodles
- some potato chips
- corn chips
- tortillas
- crisps
- crackers
- gelatin
- packet soup and quick soup
- malt extract
- applied to non-organic fruit and vegetables as a wax or pesticide
- most Asian/Chinese food (always ask the restaurant if they use it)
- some baby foods
- some cosmetics
- shampoos
- soaps and conditioners.

MSG acts as an exciter to the nervous system and can literally over-excite cells to death. Scientists use MSG to make rats obese for observation. The MSG triples the amount of insulin the pancreas produces, causing rats to become insulin resistant and obese.

It has been found to cause infertility in test animals and can cause both male and female infertility, hyperactivity, asthma, irritability, depression, mood changes, migraine, convulsions, headaches and abdominal discomfort.

Check food labels for pea, corn or whey protein as they have been hydrolysed, a process which always involves MSG.

Caffeine (in tea, green tea, coffee, chocolate, cola drinks, over the counter drugs such as painkillers) is dehydrating and stimulates the release of stress hormones. It is known to have an adverse effect on female fertility increasing the length of time it takes to conceive and increasing the risk of miscarriage and stillbirth. One study found that just 1 cup of coffee a day increases the risk of not conceiving by 55%, the risk increases with every cup of coffee you have.

In men, caffeine affects the health of sperm affecting sperm count and motility and so should be avoided by both of you.

Women who drink coffee before and during pregnancy may have twice the risk of miscarriage. This is because coffee can cross the placenta and enter the baby's underdeveloped body and organs. The baby is unable to metabolise the coffee which can lead to permanent damage. If the damage is severe, the baby may abort. Other substances which cross the placenta include alcohol, toxins in cigarettes and some drugs (both pharmaceutical and "recreational".)

Tea contains tannin which blocks the absorption of important minerals by your digestive tract.

Decaffeinated tea and coffee are not a good substitute as chemicals which are used in the decaffeination process remain in the product. De-caffeination does not remove the stimulants theobromine and theophylline and one study showed that drinking 3 cups of de-caffeinated coffee a day was associated with an increased risk of miscarriage.

If you drink a lot of coffee or tea, you can try slowly switching to decaff and then over time cutting out the decaff.   Go for plenty of water, herb or fruit teas, redbush tea, dandelion coffee, barley cup, caro or peppermint tea.

I love liquid chlorophyll in filtered water for a delicious mint flavoured, alkalising and refreshing drink.   You can buy liquid chlorophyll from Natures Sunshine.

Alcohol acts as a diuretic causing nutrients such as zinc and folic acid to be excreted. It is toxic to both the sperm and egg and the baby once you are pregnant. Ideally both partners should avoid alcohol completely as it can reduce your fertility by 50%. (A Danish study showed that drinking 7 or more alcoholic drinks a week halved the chances of getting pregnant.)

It seems that alcohol may interfere with progesterone production by the corpus luteum. It is progesterone that tells the body that a fertilised embryo is in the womb and stops the womb lining breaking down to produce a period.

Even small amounts of alcohol in pregnancy can slow down the baby's development and may lead to hyperactivity, learning difficulties and even brain damage or deafness.   The average IQ of a child affected by alcohol whilst in the womb is 20 to 80 points lower than the national average.

Sperm quality is seriously compromised by acetaldehyde, a breakdown product of alcohol. Alcohol can cause a decrease in the sperm count, the number of motile sperm and an increase in abnormal sperm.

Alcohol reduces the levels of vital sperm making hormones, so a man can wipe out his sperm count for **several months** after just one heavy drinking session. Around 80% of male alcoholics are sterile.

One study showed a lower pregnancy rate for couples where the man drank more than 10 units per week. Avoid alcoholic binges and remember the effect potentially lasts for up to 3 months.

An absolute safe limit in the pre-conception time is not known so it is better to avoid alcohol completely.

Even if you are not trying to get pregnant, it is unwise to drink more than 1 or 2 units per night for women and 2 or 3 units per night for men, and not more than once or twice per week. Remember, the average bottle of wine contains 8-10 units. 1 pint of beer = 2 units. 1 shot of spirits = 1 unit.

Sugar - pure, white and deadly! Sugar is everywhere in our food. Naturally occurring in fruits and vegetables, but also added in liberal quantities to processed foods and drinks.

Although it tastes sweet, sugar acts like an acid in the body causing damage to artery walls, interfering with brain chemistry, hormone production, promoting fat storage and disrupting blood sugar levels.

Sugar triggers the pleasure/addiction centres in the brain and the more you eat, the more you want. But sugar is destructive to the health of your body. It disrupts blood sugar control, brain chemistry and leaves an acidic residue called Advanced Glycation End products or AGEs.

These literally age your body, causing damage to the cells structure both internally in the arteries and in your skin's appearance.

The toxins produced in an acidic body reduce the absorption of proteins, minerals and other nutrients. This in turn weakens the ability to produce enzymes, hormones and other chemicals which are needed for cell energy and organ function.

When the body becomes acidic mycotoxins form. One of these is acetaldehyde, which is created from the fermentation of sugar (and the breakdown of alcohol).

Acetaldehyde reduces the absorption of vital nutrients, decreasing your ability to produce enzymes and hormones. Not only does it decrease your ability to produce enzymes, it also destroys them thereby reducing cell energy.

Acetaldehyde destroys neurotransmitters, the chemicals responsible for all nerve impulses.

Acetaldehyde binds to the walls of red blood cells, making them less flexible. This means they are less able to perform their function of getting into the capillaries of the circulatory system to transport oxygen to cells.

Acetaldehyde in the body can reduce your strength and stamina making you feel fatigued, cloud your thinking and affect both brain and nervous system functioning.

Your liver converts Acetaldehyde to alcohol depleting your body of magnesium, sulphur, hydrogen and potassium, thereby reducing cell energy. It can produce the same symptoms as being drunk, making you dizzy or mentally confused.

Eating sugary foods makes it extremely difficult for your body to maintain the correct balance of glucose circulating in your body and the correct balance of your reproductive hormones – more of this later.

Interestingly, the nutrients the body leaches to digest sugar are the key fertility nutrients such as calcium, chromium, magnesium and zinc. If you think about how much sugar we ingest just by eating processed food, eating at restaurants or snacking on chocolate and biscuits you can imagine how low our reserves of these nutrients can become.

To make matters worse, when you lose minerals your body cannot make enough digestive enzymes to break down everything you eat. This not only leads to further complications such as poor digestion and absorption of nutrients from food but it also increases your chances developing allergies and food intolerances as partly digested food particles can end up in your bloodstream.

Sugar can be hidden in foods under many different guises, but at the end of the day they're all sugar and all toxic to your system. Look out for sugar, sucrose, raw sugar, brown sugar, muscovado sugar, dextrose, honey, lactose, high fructose corn syrup, fructose, glucose, sorbitol, malitol, treacle, molasses.

6 Refined Sugar Alternatives

As with all sweeteners, use these alternatives in moderation. Any sweetening agent that gets overused can overwhelm the liver and get turned in bad fat. It's better to train your brain to avoid overly sweet foods. Syrups like maple syrup and agave syrup have some plus sides, but they are both wrought with controversy in the health community and there are better options available.

1. Stevia - A herb native to South American, stevia is 300 times sweeter than sugar. It has been used as a sweetener for centuries in South America, and in Japan, makes up 41 per cent of the sweetener market. Stevia has no calories and no glycaemic impact making it suitable for diabetics.

2. Coconut Palm Sugar - Sap from the coconut palm is heated to evaporate its water content and reduce it to usable granules. Coconut sugar is nutritious and has a low score on the glycaemic index, which means you don't get a buzz followed by a crash.

It tastes similar to brown sugar but is slightly richer. You can substitute coconut sugar for traditional sugar pretty much wherever you use the latter. Once tapped for sap, the trees can go on producing for 20 years and produce more sugar per hectare than sugar cane and benefit the local soil.

3. Xylitol – Xylitol is a natural plant sugar and can be used in place of normal sugar in drinks and cooking. It doesn't make good meringues though! It has a very low glycaemic index. In the UK it is available under the brand names Perfect Sweet and Xylobrit. The recipes in the companion recipe book "Eating to Get Pregnant" use xylitol.

4. Molasses – These are by-products of the sugar production process. Although producing sugar from sugar cane has a negative environmental impact, not

using all the products only compounds it. Because of the way traditional tabletop sugar is produced (heating the top layer which forms the crystals you have in your bowl), many of the nutritional benefits are left in the molasses. Blackstrap molasses is perhaps the most beneficial and is a good source of iron and calcium. It's quite thick and viscous and is best used in baking. It is also sweeter than sugar and so you'll need less.

5. Artichoke Syrup - Artichoke syrup is rich in inulin, a type of fiber that feeds the friendly flora of the intestinal tract. It has an exceptional sweet taste and a very low glycaemic index, making it a great sweetener for people who need to keep blood sugar levels balanced. Research indicates that the inulin found in artichoke syrup may improve gastrointestinal health and calcium absorption.

6. Lucuma Powder – Lucuma has a uniquely sweet, fragrant and subtly maple-like taste that will bring your desserts to life without making your blood sugar levels skyrocket. Lucuma is an excellent source of carbohydrates, fiber, vitamins, and minerals. It boasts of plentiful concentrations of beta-carotene, which makes lucuma a powerful immune system booster, and it is rich in iron, B2 and B1.

Its low sugar content makes it a healthy alternative to sugar for people who have diabetes and it is a great sweetener for women who are breastfeeding.

Transfats

Fat in general gets a bad name, but as you'll see later we need Essential Fatty Acids (EFAs) for our body to function properly. Unlike other members of the fat family (saturated, polyunsaturated and monounsaturated fats), trans fats, or trans-fatty acids, are largely artificial fats.

Trans fats are made by a chemical process called partial hydrogenation. Liquid vegetable oil (an otherwise healthy monounsaturated fat) is packed with hydrogen atoms and converted into a solid fat. This made what seemed an ideal fat for the food industry to work with because of its high melting point, its creamy, smooth texture and its reusability in deep-fat frying.

Partially hydrogenated fats, or trans fats, extend the shelf life of food. They also add a certain pleasing mouth-feel to all manner of processed foods. Think of buttery crackers and popcorn, crisps, biscuits, crispy French fries, chocolate, chips, pies, crunchy fish sticks, creamy frosting and melt-in-your mouth pies and pastries. All these foods owe those qualities to trans fats.

Hydrogenated fats were seen as a healthier alternative to saturated fats: using stick margarine was deemed better for you than using butter, yet numerous studies now conclude that they are actually worse.

Saturated fats raise total and bad (LDL) cholesterol levels and, crucially, they also interfere with the absorption of EFAs. Trans fats do exactly the same, but they also strip levels of good (HDL) cholesterol, the kind that helps unclog arteries. Trans fats also increase triglyceride levels in the blood, adding to our risk of cardiovascular disease.

Research shows that the chance of becoming pregnant drops by 73% for every extra 4g of trans fats (the equivalent of ½ portion of takeaway fried chicken) eaten every day! If you think how much trans fats are present in foods you might eat every day such as crisps, cakes, biscuits, chips you can see how easy it would be to overload your body with trans fats. Research shows that 80% of women with a high intake of trans fats had problems with ovulation.

Semen needs to be rich in prostaglandins which are made from EFAs, so men also need to avoid trans fats.

To minimize your consumption of trans fats be diligent about reading the ingredients and avoid the most likely culprits altogether. Trans fats are often listed as 'hydrogenated fat' or 'hardened vegetable fat' or simply 'vegetable fat.'

Processed Foods

One thing to get clear in your head is that when a food manufacturer makes a product they want it to:

1. Look good

2. Taste good

3. Be cheap to produce

4. Sell well

5. Give them maximum profits

Nutritional value, sugar, sweeteners and trans fats content are immaterial to them. They are in the business of making a product that the general public will buy repeatedly in order to sustain their money making business.

Food is not meant to come in cellophane or plastic bags, cardboard boxes, plastic bottles or tubs to be pushed into our mouths with no effort spent on preparation or proper cooking!

Next time you're in the supermarket look at the labels on products before you buy. Check for the sugar content, artificial sweeteners, trans fats, hydrogenated fats, partially hydrogenated fats, salt, high fructose corn syrup. Remember the manufacturer puts them there to disguise the use of poor quality ingredients with not just little but potentially no nutritional value at all.

Don't be deceived by products which claim to be "low sugar" or "low fat". Low sugar products generally have artificial sweeteners added and low fat products have extra sugar added to improve the taste!

I once saw a pack of liquorice which had "low in fat" emblazoned across the front – it was being offered for the shopper to taste and sure enough most of them were putting a bag into their carts.   The store employee offered me some to try, confidently telling me that the product was very healthy as it was low in fat.   "But liquorice doesn't have any fat in it" I said "and this product is 80% sugar making it an extremely unhealthy product."

The reply? "Ah, but it's low in fat!"

I'll talk a lot more about what makes a healthy diet later, but in the meantime, please for the sake of your own health and that of your unborn child, avoid processed foods.

Dairy Products

Dairy products account on average for 60-70 percent of oestrogens consumed in the diet.   We usually associate dairy and drinking milk with calcium, and never think about what else we may be consuming along with the calcium (and dairy, by the way is not the best source of calcium). Here is a list of hormones that have been found in cows' milk:

* Prolactin
* Somatostatin
* Melatonin

* Oxytocin
* Growth hormone
* Lutenizing releasing hormone
* Thyroid stimulating hormone
* Oestrogens
* Progesterone
* Insulin
* Corticosteroids and many more

Just like humans, cows produce milk when they have given birth. In order to maintain the supply of milk the cow is made pregnant again a couple of months after having their calf.   It continues to be milked whilst pregnant and all the cows pregnancy hormones go into their milk and other dairy products.

Extended periods of milking can give a cow mastitis, so they're given anti-biotics which also end up in their milk.

Consumption of milk has been linked to certain cases of male infertility. Excess oestrogen and pesticide exposure has been linked to PCOS and Endometriosis. Studies have found higher concentrations of pesticides in cheese than in non-organically grown fruit and vegetables.

Minimise your intake of animal products as they have a high content of hormones, pesticides and herbicides which are known endocrine disruptors. They play havoc with your hormones and this can stop you ovulating.

If you must have milk, organic sheep or goats milk may be a better option as they are less intensively produced. There's a trend toward having skimmed or light milk which has had the fat removed from it. Unfortunately, this means that the fat soluble vitamins A, D and E which are essential for reproductive health are also removed.

In my view, the only acceptable dairy product is organic, plain live or bio yogurt as it contains bacteria which are beneficial to your gut. Avoid fruit yogurts as they can contain as much as 8 teaspoons of sugar. The live bacteria feed on the sugar, and when the sugar runs out, the bacteria die off!

Don't be fooled by the "friendly bacteria" drinks and yogurts which are all the rage at the moment. You'd need to drink around a bath tub full to get as many of the good bacteria as you'll get from a good quality acidophilus supplement.

We tend to be brainwashed from an early age that we need to drink milk for the calcium content. You need to bear in mind that cow's milk is intended for cows not humans. It's designed to meet the nutritional needs of a growing calf and the calcium content is bound up with a protein called casein, (a component of wood glue) which we don't have the correct enzymes to digest.

For humans, better sources of calcium are vegetables, sesame and sunflower seeds, hazel nuts, brazil nuts, almonds and chickpeas.

Wheat products

For many of us a diet without wheat or bread is unthinkable. I've been conducting Food Intolerance Tests on patients for nearly 15 years now and find that the vast majority of people who have problems with their digestion are intolerant to either wheat or dairy or both.

The incidence of Coeliac disease is increasing, most people know someone who suffers from this condition and it's estimated to affect 1 in 100 people. But there are even more people who are, without knowing it, intolerant to wheat.

So, what's the difference between a wheat allergy as in Coeliac disease and wheat intolerance?

With an <u>allergy</u> the reaction is immediate. The typical symptoms are:

Hives, (Urticaria), rashes, swelling, vomiting, palpitations, blushing, difficulty breathing, sudden tiredness, stomach cramps, rapid drop in blood pressure.

With an <u>intolerance</u> the reaction can be delayed – up to 24 to 48 hours later. The typical symptoms are:

Itching, sinus problems, bloating, anaemia, diarrhoea or constipation, Crohn's disease, IBS, diverticulitis, depression, brain fog, poor concentration, dark circles under the eyes, headaches.

Humans have only been eating wheat for around 10,000 years. Before then we were hunter gatherers, eating fish and meat, fruits and vegetables. If you were to condense the whole of human history into 24 hours, we would have been eating grains for, at most, 6 minutes.

We have not really evolved to digest the gluten in grains, in particular gliadin which is found in wheat. Rye and barley contain a form of gluten similar to gliadin and many people who are intolerant to wheat also have a problem with these grains.

Gliadin is known to irritate the lining of the gut, it can create holes in the gut wall which allow undigested particles of food to leak into the bloodstream. This can give rise to a whole range of problems, which at first glance would seem unrelated to what you eat.

If your digestion is weak you can retain gliadorphins in the blood. These are wheat-based opioids which can make you crave the very wheat products you are allergic to!

Many people's diets are heavily dependent on wheat. I've seen people who have a wheat based cereal for breakfast, sandwiches for lunch, pasta for dinner and wonder why they feel rubbish.

You need to think carefully about the amount of wheat in your diet, particularly if you're in the habit of eating white bread. Nutritionally it is of zero value and it has the potential to cause you serious health problems.

The main problem with buying refined white flour products is that they are made using wheat strains with a very high gluten content. This is done to speed up commercial bread making which is great for the manufacturer but not for you.

If you really can't manage without a sandwich for lunch, then do at least make sure that your breakfast and dinner (and all snacks in between) are wheat free. Also have a wholegrain bread, or try having a wrap or flatbread.

Food intolerances

If you're not sure if you have a food intolerance, just answer these questions:

- ☐ Are you chronically tired?
- ☐ Can you gain weight in hours?
- ☐ Do you get bloated after you've eaten?
- ☐ Do you suffer from diarrhoea or constipation?
- ☐ Do you get stomach pains or cramps?
- ☐ Do you ever feel really sleepy after eating?
- ☐ Are you sinuses congested, or do you have sneezing or a runny nose?
- ☐ Do you have rashes, itching, asthma or shortness of breath?

- ☐ Do you get colds a lot?
- ☐ Do you have water retention?
- ☐ Do you suffer from migraines or headaches?
- ☐ Do you get aches and pains from time to time, particularly after you've eaten certain foods?
- ☐ Do you get spells of depression for no apparent reason?
- ☐ Do you lose concentration or get brain fog?
- ☐ Do you notice you feel better if you have a complete change of diet – for instance when on holiday?

If you answered yes to any of these questions, it's possible that you have a food intolerance. If you answered yes to 4 or more then it's pretty much a dead certainty.

You don't have to rely on guesswork to work out if you have a food intolerance. There are very reliable blood tests available which look for IgG antibodies in the blood. Go to http://www.yorktest.com/ for more information.

Food Intolerance and anti-sperm antibodies.

The link between food intolerances and anti-sperm antibodies is now well established. Studies have found that women with multiple allergies and food intolerances were more likely to miscarry.

An overactive immune system is more likely to attack its own body cells. From an immunological point of view an embryo and sperm cell are foreign bodies. But Mother Nature was clever; she programmed our immune systems to distinguish between an everyday invader and a sperm cell or embryo.

A normal and healthy immune response to an embryo or sperm cell is orchestrated by Th2 cytokines. They suppress your killer cells (that's what they are called) to leave the embryo unharmed.

Because of this protection many pregnant women are poor wound healers and can come down really badly with a cold or flu. Your natural protection has been suppressed so that your baby can develop properly.
An abnormal immune response to the implantation of the fertilized egg is orchestrated by Th1 cytokines. Rather than suppressing your killer cells they stimulate their activity. This can lead to defects and the loss of the fetus.

The two most widely spread food intolerances are gluten and dairy. Since most people have some level of allergy to gluten and/or dairy, and for all the reasons above, it's advisable to avoid gluten and dairy altogether during the preconception and pregnancy period.

Cola/Soda

Fizzy drinks contain a vast array of chemicals, phosphoric acid, sugar, sweeteners, caffeine and preservatives. They are toxic to your body, leaching vital nutrients from your system including calcium.

Don't be fooled by "diet" or caffeine free colas. If it's a cola you should view it as a potential poison to your body.

Think back to the chemistry lessons you did at school. If you have an excess of acid in your body, you need an alkaline substance to neutralise it. Your body gets that alkaline in the form of calcium from your bones. Sadly, we have a generation of young people who are at risk of developing osteoporosis in their twenties, due to high consumption of soda drinks.

We tend to take it for granted now that fizzy drinks are the drink of choice for many of us and are seen as being perfectly acceptable. But research suggests that they can cause weight gain and long-term health problems if drunk every day for as little as a month.

The research, by Bangor University and published in the European Journal Of Nutrition, reported that soft drinks actually alter metabolism, so that our muscles use sugar for energy instead of burning fat.

It seems that exposure to liquid sugar causes genes in our muscles to change their behaviour, perhaps permanently. Not only do we pile on weight, but our metabolism becomes less efficient and less able to cope with rises in blood sugar, say the researchers. This, in turn, increases the risk of type 2 diabetes.

Research published by the American Heart Association warned that men who drink a standard 12oz can of sugar-sweetened beverage every day have a 20 per cent higher risk of heart disease compared to men who don't drink any sugar-sweetened drinks.

The study suggested this may be a result of the sugar rush these soft drinks cause. This increased sudden sugar load on the body may also explain research which found just two carbonated drinks (330ml each) every week appears to double the risk of pancreatic cancer.

In children, soft drinks have been linked to addict-like cravings, as well as twisting kids' appetites so they hunger for junk food. Researchers at University College London's Health Behaviour Research Centre discovered a powerful — and lucrative — effect sugary soft drinks have on youngsters.

The study of 346 children aged around 11 found drinking soft drinks makes them want to drink more often, even when they're not actually thirsty — and that their preference is for more sugary drinks.

Children who drank water or fruit juice in the tests didn't show this unnecessary need to drink. The researchers expressed concern that this may set the children's habits for life — in particular, giving them an 'increased preference for sweet things in the mouth', without compensating for the extra calories by eating less food.

More recent research suggests fizzy drinks may sway children's tastes towards high-calorie, high-salt food. The researchers said this wasn't about simple fussiness. Instead, our tastes for food and drink seem to be shaped in a like-with-like manner.

The bottom line is that sugary, fizzy drinks (and so called diet drinks) are to be avoided if you have PCOS and if you want to get pregnant.

Tap Water

The most important single change you can make to improve your diet and health is to drink at least 3 pints of fresh water every day.

Your body is composed of roughly 80% water. You need on average, 3 pints of plain water every day to replace lost body fluids and maintain a healthy system. That is 3 pints of water on top of whatever tea, coffee, fruit juice or other drinks you consume.

It may sound a lot, but if you aim to drink a glass of water every hour or so, it is easy to drink the minimum recommended amount. You need to bear in mind that if you are very active or you exercise a lot you will need to drink more water.

Many people believe that drinking tea and coffee all day is not a problem and that they are getting plenty of fluid. However, what they don't realise is that tea, coffee, cocoa, and cola drinks all contain caffeine.

Caffeine acts as a diuretic, that is, it makes you pass more urine. So the net result is that your body has not had the fluid which it needs. It is recommended by many health advisors that you should drink one glass of water for every cup of tea or coffee that you drink.

If you do not drink enough water you will gradually become dehydrated. Your body will divert water away from non essential areas to those which are essential. If you skin is very dry, or your joints are getting creaky this may be a sign that you are dehydrated!

Sadly it's a fact that waterways in most parts of the world are regularly polluted by some level of industrial waste and by-products, pharmaceutical drugs, pesticides and herbicides and commercial cleaning products.

Heavy metals are the most common of the toxins reaching our water supply through industrial waste, jet fuel exhaust residue and a variety of other sources.

Pharmaceutical drugs are commonly found in tap water. In the Us as many as 74% of the population takes prescription drugs. Because the drugs do not metabolize fully, small quantities are excreted via faeces and urine and flushed away.

Toilet water is often treated and filtered before being discharged into lakes and rivers thereby re-entering the water supply. The trouble is, many drugs are not filtered out via the regular filtration process.

Minute quantities of chemotherapy drugs, contraceptive pills, antidepressants, anxiolitics, anabolic steroids, HRT (hormone replacement therapy), heart drugs etc. have been found in tap water.

It's become almost a fashion statement to carry round a plastic bottle of water everywhere you go. Do be aware that plastics leach chemicals into the water which are not good for you.

Watch out for flavoured waters, they often contain sugar and/or artificial sweeteners and flavourings. If you want to flavour your water then squeeze the juice of a fresh orange, lemon or lime into it for a wholly natural drink.

To make sure your drinking water is clean and health giving, either use a jug water filter or ideally install a plumbed in water filter at home. When you are out of the house carry your water in a glass bottle.

GENERAL LIFESTYLE & ENVIRONMENTAL FACTORS

Anything wrapped in plastic!

If you buy from your local supermarket, chances are that some of your fruit and vegetables will be shrink wrapped in plastic. Soft plastics contain xenoestrogens (artificial hormones) which leak into the food and disrupt your own hormone levels. Buy your fruit and vegetables fresh and make sure that there is no soft plastic on them. The same goes for any food such as cheese, wrapped in a soft plastic. Also, avoid the use of cling film for the same reason.

Bisphenol A is a synthetic oestrogen used in the manufacture of many food containers, baby bottles and cans. One study showed that women who had a history of miscarriage had 3 times the levels of bisphenol A as women who had never miscarried. Male workers who inhaled the dust from this product developed breasts – such is the influence of the oestrogen content.

Avoid drinking out of plastic water bottles, storing your food in plastic food wrappers, wearing surgical gloves, buying products in food wrap and touching printing ink with your hands. What do all these have in common?

Soft plastics contain Phthalates and PVC. Which are known endocrine disruptors and estrogen mimickers, linked to asthma, negative developmental and birth defects, immune system dysfunction, endometriosis and infertility.

Cans and plastic bottles of fizzy drinks contain 6 times the amount of aluminium compared to the same drinks in glass bottles. Don't buy water in a plastic bottle, especially if it has been exposed to heat.

Electro Magnetic Radiation

Because we live in a high tech age we are subjected to electro magnetic radiation on a daily basis. Realistically it's impossible to completely avoid it, but you do need to take whatever steps you can to minimise exposure.

Electro magnetic radiation is potentially damaging to your own health and that of your unborn child.

Mobile phones

20 years ago it was rare to see someone with a mobile phone and if you did they were almost the size of a house brick! Nowadays, it seems that they are a compulsory "must have" accessory for everyone, including children.

Mobile phones transmit and receive radiation at frequencies between 825 and 915 megahertz (MHz). These radio waves are emitted by both mobile phone handsets and base stations.

This radiation has the ability to heat human tissue, similar to the way in which microwave ovens heat food. This heat can cause live tissue and cells to die.

Children in particular are vulnerable to phone radiation. Some studies have shown that mobile phone radiation can cause damage to the DNA of cells – there was damage to chromosomes, changes to the activity of certain genes, and an increase in the rate of cell division and replication.

This is potentially catastrophic to a developing foetus. Many studies also link mobile phone use with decrease in production and quality of a man's sperm. I'm also aware of young males who habitually carried a mobile phone in their trouser pocket developing testicular cancer.

If you must be contactable 24/7, then carry your phone away from your body in a bag or briefcase. Use a headset so that you don't have to hold the phone to your ear. Never carry your phone on your person in a pocket, especially near to your heart or ovaries.

Cordless phones

Cordless phones emit the same type of radiation as mobile phones. However, it seems that the base station is the main problem as it emits the same type of radiation as a mobile phone station tower. Depending on the model you have, it might be more than twice the amount of radiation as mobile phone tower.

The best way to avoid exposure to cordless phone radiation is to not have one in your home or office. Use a standard fixed line and location phone instead- this is especially important if you are working to overcome fertility problems and/or miscarriages and want to have the healthiest possible baby.

If it's unavoidable for you to use a cordless phone, use it as infrequently as you can. Move the base station as far away from the areas that you use the most as you can.

Wireless technology

Wireless internet, computer networks and hot-spots as well as wireless mice, keyboards and speakers, also operate by using radio frequency non-ionising radiation similar to that used by mobile and cordless phones.

Studies have shown that the radiation from these devices can damage DNA, our self repairing mechanisms and disrupt the blood-brain barrier (allowing toxins and pathogens to reach the brain). It may also lead to lowered immunity, decreased melatonin levels, cell damage, formation of micronuclei, changes in calcium metabolism affecting communication between cells, changes in brainwave patterns as seen on EEG's, plus effects observed on many different systems of the body. Although there are still no long term studies on the effects of exposure to the radiation emitted by wireless technologies, it is estimated the results will be very similar to those discussed previously, linked to mobile and cordless phone use.

Electric Blankets

Electric blankets have been seen to produce electromagnetic radiation over 70,000 times higher than normal acceptable levels. The electromagnetic radiation produced by electric blankets is able to penetrate about 6-7 inches (close to 20cm) into the body. Studies have shown that the use of electric blankets has been linked to an increase in the incidence and development of childhood leukaemia.

The use of electric blankets have also been linked to an increased rate of miscarriage, impaired baby development, increased stress levels, memory problems and possibly other types of cancers.

Microwaved food.

Leaving aside the fact that microwave ovens give out electro-magnetic radiation within a range of 15 feet and through brick walls - microwaving food destroys its vitamin content; damages the cell walls of food to such a degree that the remaining particles are barely recognisable as food by the gut, causing immune response reactions.

Carcinogenic toxins could be leached from plastic or paper plates or covers and mix with your food. If you bear in mind that many people use processed pre-prepared quick foods in their microwaves, it is easy to imagine that far from feeding the body, the food they eat is potentially highly toxic to the body.

Microwave ovens produce micro wavelength radiation of 2450 Mega Hertz (MHz) or 2.45 Giga Hertz (GHz). This radiation passes though the molecules of your food.

They emit a form of EM energy similar to radio and light waves, which are used to relay TV programs, long distance phone calls and communicate with satellites

Just as a magnet has a positive and negative polarity, so do the molecules of our bodies and our food molecules. The microwaves cause the poles in the molecules to rotate millions of times over. This 'polarity rotation' generates heat (which makes the food hot) but, in the process it also damages the molecules and the surrounding molecules breaking and tearing them apart. Essentially deforming them and making them not just useless but dangerous to the body.

As long ago as 1989, doctors began to study the effects of microwaving food on both the food itself and the human body. It began to emerge that every microwave oven leaks electromagnetic radiation, harms food and converts nutrients to dangerous and toxic carcinogens. A study published in 1992 showed that people who ate microwaved food had lower levels of haemoglobin, higher levels of LDL cholesterol, and lower levels of immune cells.

Russian research, concluded that microwaved food had 60-90% decrease in nutritional value, and there was a decreased bio-availability of vitamins B, C, E, essential minerals and fatty acids. The term "microwave sickness" was coined as the changes to the blood, described above, leads to a variety of symptoms and conditions including reproductive problems and cancer.

Here are the key reasons for NEVER eating microwaved food:

Vitamins, minerals and nutrients become altered and useless to the human body. When trying to conceive and during pregnancy it's crucial that your body gets all the nutrients it needs.

1. Regular eating of microwaved food alters and can shut down male and female hormone production. Altered hormone production can lead to poor egg and sperm health, inability to conceive and miscarriages.

2. The human body can not break down and absorb microwaved "nutrients" and their toxic by-products.
3. The effects of microwaved food by-products on the body are long lasting.
4. Vegetables and meat proteins are altered and turned into carcinogenic compounds.
5. Ingestion of microwaved food has been linked to stomach and intestinal cancer and tumours, loss of memory, concentration, decrease in intelligence, emotional instability and infertility.

BHA and BHT (E320 and E321)

These are food additives used for preserving fat and they are blamed for birth defects, infertility and cancer.

Found in bacon, foods containing artificial colours and flavours, baked goods, canned food, powdered soups, instant mashed potatoes, edible oil, margarine, gum, reduced fat spreads, baby oil and baby lotion, lipstick, eyeliner, shaving cream, plastic food wraps containing polyethylene.

BHA & BHT can cause fatigue, hyperactivity, asthma, cancer, birth defects, infertility, dermatitis, skin blistering, extreme weakness, eye irritation, weakened immune system and allergic reactions in aspirin-sensitive people.

Like MSG this is an additive which keeps finding its way into our food, cosmetics and personal care products in spite of the known health dangers.

Check labels and ideally avoid process foods completely.

Smoking

Smoking can bring on an early menopause, decrease sperm count, make sperm sluggish and increase the number of abnormal sperm.

If either of you are smokers and you are serious about getting pregnant, you need to stop NOW. (Acupuncture treatment can help with this.)

Smoking damages the reproductive system of both men and women. Smoking affects hormone balance by making FSH levels significantly higher than they should be. It has the affect of ageing your eggs, affects the womb lining, reducing the chances of pregnancy and increasing the risk of miscarriage, low birth weight, prematurity and birth defects.

Passive smoking also affects a woman's chances of conception. It can bring on irregular periods and early menopause by lowering oestrogen levels. It depletes the body of Vitamin C and zinc, increases the risk of miscarriage and halves the chances of you getting pregnant. For women smokers, the effect has been compared to an increase in female age of more than 10 years.

For men smoking affects erectile function, sperm count, motility and morphology and can make smokers 75% less fertile than non-smokers. It affects the DNA of the sperm leading to increased risk of miscarriage and affects the health of the unborn child.

Smoking for either partner almost halves the success rate of IVF, ICSI or IUI. These risks are the same if you actively or passively smoke, so both partners must stop.

Use of Tampons

Tampons may affect the natural balance of vaginal secretions and cervical mucus. Tampons may have as many as 400 chemicals and bleach in them. There are suggestions that tampon use is implicated in the increasing incidence of endometriosis and polycystic ovaries.

Menstrual blood is meant to flow away and be eliminated from the body. Holding it in place with a tampon can create stagnation and clotty menstrual blood.

If you don't want to use sanitary towels, there are alternatives such as the mooncup which has the advantage of being washable and re-usable. Visit the mooncup website (http://www.mooncup.co.uk) and watch the video for more reasons to stop using tampons!

Environmental Toxins

Exposure to environmental toxins (in the form of industrial chemicals) both in utero and neonatally can damage your fertility. Most chemicals used in everyday life don't go through the same checks medicines do. Consequently, poisonous chemicals end up circulating in our environment, food supply, air and water.

The strongest evidence of heavy metal and environmental pollution adversely interfering with reproductive function in women has been found for lead. Sperm are more sensitive to heavy metals and industrial pollutants than eggs. Many sperm abnormalities are linked to these toxins. The majority of these chemicals are found in the atmosphere, on the ground in cities and in the waterways.

Do what you can to avoid or eliminate these environmental toxins:

Pesticides found on non-organic fruit and vegetables, meat, dairy products and unfiltered tap water.

Formaldehyde in air fresheners, deodorants, floor polish, upholstery cleaners

Bisphenols found in plastic containers and which leach into food and water

Organic solvents used in paints, varnishes, lacquers, adhesives, glues, and degreasing/cleaning agents, and in the production of dyes, polymers, plastics, textiles, printing inks, agricultural products, and pharmaceuticals.

<u>Paint fumes and perfumes</u>

<u>Dry-cleaning chemicals</u>

Studies have found that exposure to chlorinated hydrocarbons (e.g., DDT, PCB, pentachlorophenol, hexachlorocyclohexane) has been associated with an increase in rates of miscarriage and endometriosis.

Recreational and Over the Counter Drugs

In women, marijuana use can cause irregular periods and prevent ovulation.

Men who smoke marijuana have less seminal fluid, a reduced sperm count and sperm which swim very fast, but too early, reducing their chances of fertilisation. It lowers libido and cot death has been linked to marijuana use.

Cocaine use damages all the semen parameters and its effects can be seen in the sperm for up to 2 years after use. Sperm count is lowered, sperm move poorly and there are higher than average levels of abnormal sperm. Heroin reduces testosterone levels.

If cocaine and heroin are taken together by a woman it will make it harder for her to conceive, she is more likely to miscarry or have a child with a malformation.

Cocaine can result in neurological damage to the baby. Recreational drug users should ideally avoid all drugs for at least a year before conception.

Over the Counter drugs can interfere with your fertility affecting the production of FSH, LH and the functioning of the pituitary gland. Some interfere with the production of healthy sperm or decrease sperm motility.

If you or your partner takes sleeping pills, anti-histamines, anti-biotic long term, tranquillisers or painkillers then you should discuss their impact on your fertility with your doctor.

Stress

It's important to exercise, eat well and keep stress levels down at all times, but particularly when you are trying for a baby. The stress hormones (adrenalin and cortisol) are released when your brain thinks that you are in some kind of danger. This is an automatic response to any anxious thought. Adrenalin release is not under the control of your conscious mind and so you must begin to be aware of your thoughts and what makes you feel stressed.

Too much cortisol in your bloodstream can interfere with your hormone balance and the production of your reproductive hormones.

If you are constantly worrying about whether or not you will get pregnant, about work or your relationship, your brain will release stress hormones. The major problem for you is that when your body makes hormones, it's a bit like baking cakes. In the same way that you might take flour, sugar and butter and decide to make a sponge cake or a fruit cake, so from the basic ingredients (i.e. food) your body can choose to make reproductive hormones or stress hormones. Stress hormones will always take priority and so your reproductive hormones suffer.

Excess stress hormones can affect your periods, egg quality, sperm quality in men and increase the risk of miscarriage.

It's important that you learn to manage your stress. You might find my book Stop Stressing Start Living a useful tool. It will teach you how to reduce stress symptoms and comes with guided relaxations. Learning to control your breath and relax is key to switching off the stress response and production of stress hormones. For more information visit Amazon.

It's important to keep a sense of balance in your life. As I said earlier, sex should not be just about baby making, but an expression of your love and commitment to each other. Make sure you have relaxation time together and that you do things you enjoy. Build a strong and supportive relationship between you, you'll need it when you're pregnant and parents of a baby that seems to take over your whole life!

Make sure you don't put your life on hold while you're waiting to get pregnant. I've talked to many couples who are "living in the future" and forget that the only reality is the present moment in time. I often recommend to couples that they go and do all the things that they won't be able to do when they have children. It might be exotic holidays, spontaneous breaks away or nights out. The key thing is to come back to the present, appreciate what you have right now and make being with your partner a fulfilling and rich existence NOW.

I often relate the experience of a friend of mine. She had one child and was desperate to have a second. She put off going back to work because she was going to get pregnant soon. She didn't join a gym or resume some of her outside hobbies and activities. Every month she charted her fertility and did her ovulation tests.

The months and years ticked by and she didn't get pregnant again. Finally, she gave up, got a great job she loved, joined the gym and did all the things she'd put on hold. Within 6 months she was pregnant!

Work Patterns can be a major source of stress.

Research shows that people in high stress jobs are more at risk of miscarriage. However, if you work shifts or you have irregular work patterns this can lead to the production of stress hormones, affect your sleep patterns and your general health.

If this applies to you then it's vitally important that you take steps to alleviate your stress as much as possible. Make sure that you leave work at work and don't bring it home with you. Take time to relax and do things you enjoy and get plenty of sleep.

Exercise

Exercise is a great way to burn off stress hormones and will be good to improve muscle tone, blood, nutrient and oxygen flow to your uterus and ovaries and to the testes.

It's important to make sure you're doing the right amount of exercise. Quality and quantity are really important here. You want to keep your body active, strong and supple but you don't want to train 7 days a week and exhaust yourself. Exercising for more than 15 hours a week can affect and inhibit ovulation and sperm production.

The key is to do what you enjoy and get a balance of cardiovascular exercise (makes your heart beat faster), resistance exercise (to build strength) and stretching to keep you supple.

Finding an exercise that you enjoy is important, because then you're more likely to keep it up. It can be as simple as a brisk 20 minute walk every day with a friend, playing badminton, doing a Zumba class or going dancing.

I like Zumba as it's fun and helps build strength and stamina. Pilates is particularly good for strengthening the core muscles and I highly recommend it. Yoga is excellent for strength and suppleness.

A couple of words of caution about swimming and cycling. If you enjoy swimming then do incorporate it into your exercise routine. Just be aware that pools are generally heavily chlorinated and make sure that you don't swallow any water. Try not to stay in the pool too long as chlorine will be absorbed through the skin, 20 minutes is plenty.

If you choose to cycle, stay away from busy roads so that you're not breathing in heavily polluted air which will challenge your system to eliminate toxins. For men, use an ergonomically designed saddle which will not compress the testicles. Studies show that sperm counts are reduced in men who cycle frequently.

Most importantly, do what you enjoy and not what you think you should be doing.

CREATING HEALTHY EGGS AND SPERM

It takes 150 days to mature an egg and 100 days to produce sperm. Within that time you have a golden opportunity to improve the health of your eggs and sperm and so increase both the chances of conceiving, and going on to have a healthy baby.

I always say to clients when we talk about diet that they need to think about dietary changes in terms of creating vibrant health for the rest of their lives, not just to get pregnant.

Most of the diseases in the modern world are a result of our highly acidic, processed food diet. We've moved far away from the diets of our ancestors which contained fresh, natural foods to consuming "food" that has been processed so much that it's more toxic than nourishing.

It's no wonder that arthritis, heart disease, cancer, osteoporosis and diabetes are so prevalent. For many couples their fertility problems can be traced back to an acidic diet leading to an acidic internal state.

The human body should be slightly alkaline in order to function properly. Acidity and alkalinity are measured on the PH scale of 1 to 14. A measurement below 7 indicates acidity in the body and we're aiming for a measurement of 7.4.   (You can get test sticks to measure the acidity/alkalinity of your urine or saliva on Amazon – just search for PH test strips.)

Cervical secretions need to be alkaline for sperm to survive and for a fertilised embryo to embed. Excess oestrogens from the diet are converted into acid waste compounding the problems caused by an acidic diet. Permanently high oestrogen levels lead to hormone imbalances which are seen as heavy periods, endometriosis, PMS and low sperm counts.

A fertility boosting diet needs to contain all the vital food groups – carbohydrates, fibre, essential fats, protein and water *in the right proportions.* You need to aim for 80% of your food intake being alkaline and no more than 20% acid in nature.

All living foods (animal or plant) are influenced by the environment in which they grow and the processes they are subjected to before they reach your plate. In order for your body to function at its best and stay healthy, it needs high quality food.

As long ago as 1936, warnings were being given about the poor quality of soil and its effect on crops. Problems have arisen because chemical fertilisers primarily contain the growth promoting elements nitrogen and phosphorus and exclude the trace elements which are vital to human health.

It follows that if the soil does not contain essential minerals, then plants cannot take them up. In 1991 a report showed that the mineral content of our food was over 45% greater in 1946 than in 1991.

If your budget will run to it, eat organic fruit and vegetables and organic/free range meat and fish. If you have the space to grow your own fruit and veggies – even better, nothing compares to picking salad leaves or tomatoes and having them on your plate within 10 minutes.

So, which foods are acid and which are alkaline? As a general rule of thumb, vegetables and salad vegetables are alkaline. Soft fruits with a high sugar content, tend to be more acid and animal proteins are acid. Grains and bread are acid in nature and of course, processed, microwaved foods are highly acid.

If you want to read a full discussion of the PH of foods, I recommend The PH Miracle by Dr. Robert O Young and Shelley Redford Young. (Available from Amazon.)

You'll find the guidelines in this book and the Eating to Get Pregnant recipe book fall within the broad guidelines given in The PH Miracle.

DETOXING

The first step is to start detoxing your body. It's no good starting to bring in healthy foods if you're still putting rubbish into your body. Go back to the previous section and re-read the information about toxic foods if you need to.

When I see a couple for the first time I always ask them to complete a diet diary for a week so I can get a handle on their normal eating patterns. It's amazing how many times they come in and say they hadn't realised how bad their diet was till they started to write it down. Sometimes people are quite embarrassed to hand over their diet diary because they know it's bad.

When you've decided to eat a healthier diet, one of the biggest challenges can be overcoming your cravings or addictions to unhealthy food. Some people really give themselves a hard time about it, but it's important to realize that a lot of the most addictive foods have emotional connections in your brain that have been wired there for years.

If you've been eating certain junk foods for 5 years, then potentially it's going to be difficult to break that habit. Don't beat yourself up if you don't succeed in 2 weeks. Most junk foods are engineered to be as addictive as possible. Coca Cola actually contained cocaine (hence the name) when it was first released in America, until cocaine was banned.

While there are no illegal addictive substances in today's junk foods, there are still many legal addictive ingredients used. Sugar is probably the worst ingredient added to many so called "foods".

The first thing to do when you want to curb your cravings is get a reality check on what you actually eat.

Researchers were startled when they found that almost every diet program that worked had one thing that other diet programs didn't: Their participants kept a diet diary. Subsequent research has shown that just keeping a diet diary without consciously trying to change the food intake resulted in lost weight.

Keeping a diet diary brings you face to face with your food choices. Without a diet diary, it can be so easy to fool yourself that your diet isn't too bad. But when you look at your diary and see you've had 5 bags of crisps/chips or bars of candy that week, the evidence is undeniable.

At the end of the week, take a look at your eating habits. Were they what you expected? Did you eat more or less of certain foods than you expected?

Once you've got your reality check on what your diet is really like, you can decide how you're going to eliminate the junk foods that you craved. For some people, the reality check is such a shock that they immediately eliminate all sugary, processed, junk foods.

For some people going "cold turkey" feels like too much of a challenge. If you've been eating one microwave dinner a day for the last 3 years, don't try to just dump it for life immediately.

Instead, pick a percentage. Say, 50%. For the next month, you'll cut your consumption of microwave dinners by 50%. The month after that, you can reduce it to just once a week. Finally, you can quit entirely.

This allows you to cut down on your intake of junk foods while still fulfilling some of the cravings. It makes the whole process a lot easier.

As you make changes, keep on with your diet diary, so that you can also see your achievements right there on paper. Anytime you eat healthy foods, you can flip back through those pages and feel good about your progress.

According to Steven Covey, author of "Seven Habits of Highly Effective People," it takes about 30 days for a habit to become ingrained.

Developing the diet diary habit might be difficult for the first week or two. But once you've got the habit down, it'll virtually run on autopilot from then on.

When you get started on eliminating the junk from your diet, you've obviously got to replace it with something else. First, let's look at what happens to your blood sugar levels when you eat a highly processed diet.

BALANCING YOUR BLOOD SUGAR LEVELS

Whether you're trying to lose weight, improve fertility, control diabetes or alleviate the symptoms of PCOS, it's important to be aware of the effects of the sugar in carbohydrates on your body and in particular, your blood sugar level.

Carbohydrates provide fuel for your body to burn for energy. However, processed foods are often heavily laden with carbohydrates which release their sugar content very quickly and have a detrimental effect on your health.

In an ideal world, we want to see the level of sugar circulating in the bloodstream to be fairly stable throughout the day, supplying our energy needs. If we were to plot this on a chart, we'd want it to look something like this:

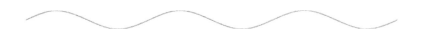

The highs and lows correspond to the amount of sugar in the bloodstream, depending on whether you've just eaten or are getting hungry.

When you eat a carbohydrate with a fast releasing, high sugar content, the level of sugar in the blood stream rises sharply.

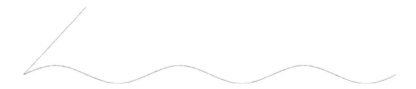

When there is too much sugar in the bloodstream, your pancreas releases insulin, taking the surplus sugar out of the blood and dumping it in fat stores. The more sugar there is in the blood, the more insulin is released and this can cause the blood sugar level to fall too low and you get hungry.

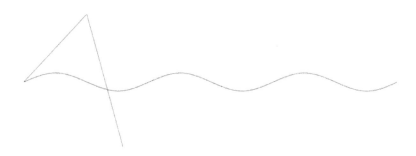

This is when many people will reach for a sugary snack or drink to give them a boost of energy. This works for a brief period, until more insulin is released and their energy dips again. And yes, you've guessed it, they eat another high carb snack or meal. So they can end up with the blood sugar level yo yo-ing throughout the day.

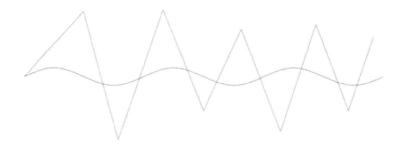

Ultimately, this can lead to a situation where your body becomes "insulin resistant" that is, it ignores the insulin instruction to dump excess sugar into fat stores and levels can become dangerously high. This leads to Type 2 diabetes, which is becoming more and more common.

Women with PCOS are often prescribed the drug metformin, used in Type 2 diabetes, to try and control their blood sugar level. However, you can do a lot with your diet to regain that important control.

Answer the questions in this quiz to find out how well you are managing your blood sugar levels:

1. Do you feel you need more than 7 hours sleep each night?
2. Do you feel sluggish or lethargic in the morning?

3. Do you need a caffeine drink such as tea, coffee, cola to get you going in the morning?
4. Do you drink caffeinated drinks regularly through the day?
5. Do you need to pass water frequently?
6. Do you have sweaty palms?
7. Do you smoke cigarettes or cigars?
8. Do you have an alcoholic drink most evenings?
9. Do you have a thirst that is not quenched by drinking water?
10. Do you feel sleepy during the day?
11. Do you crave chocolates, cakes, biscuits or bread through the day?
12. Are you too tired to exercise?
13. Do you lose concentration at times?
14. Do you get irritable or dizzy if you don't eat often?

If you answered yes to 3 or more questions, it's likely that your body is struggling to control blood sugar levels. It's important that you take heed of the advice in this book if you are to avoid problems. If you answered yes to 5 or more questions, you really must change your diet and eating patterns. If there is no improvement in your symptoms, it would be advisable for you to consult your doctor.

Back in 1981, the Glycaemic Index (GI) was invented by Dr Thomas Wolever and Dr David Jenkins at the University of Toronto. The GI is a ranking of carbohydrates on a scale from 0 to 100 according to the extent to which they raise blood sugar levels after eating. Foods with a high GI are those which are rapidly digested and absorbed and result in marked fluctuations in blood sugar levels. So the GI tells us about the quality of a carbohydrate.

Sugar has a GI value of 100 and other foods are measured against that. People were advised to eat mainly foods with a low GI (55 or less), or moderate GI value (56 -69). It was suggested that high GI value foods (70+) should be combined with a low GI value food, or avoided altogether.

Here are some examples of GI values:

FOOD	GI
Burgen mixed grain bread	34
Muffin	54
Special K cereal	54
Cola drink	63
Croissant	67

Weetabix	69
Wholemeal bread	69
Crumpet	69
Bagel	69
Swede	72
Watermelon	72
Gluten free bread	79
Cornflakes	84
Puffed wheat	89
Rice milk	92

So you can see that Muffins, Special K were considered fine to eat. Cola, croissants, bagels were fine in moderation whereas watermelon was in the "to be avoided" group.

The big problem with only looking at how fast the sugar content of a food hits the blood stream, is that it takes no account of just how much sugar there is in the food. Because some foods typically have a low carbohydrate content, Harvard researchers created the GL rating system that takes into account the amount of carbohydrates in a given serving of a food.

The GL looks at both the *quality* of the sugar - how fast it releases, and the *quantity*. The GL means the total "Glycaemic Load" on the body. It's worked out by using a simple formula. Take the GI value of a food, multiply it by the amount of carbohydrate in a food and divide by 100.

So, why is this important? First, let me explain that if you want to keep blood sugar levels stable, return your body to an alkaline state, improve your fertility, maintain your ideal weight and enjoy good health, you need to aim for each of your 3 main meals having a GL value of 15.

If you want to lose weight, then you'd aim for each of the 3 main meals having a GL value of 10. In order to keep blood sugar levels stable through the day, you'd add in 2 snacks mid morning and afternoon, each with a GL value of 5.

When we add the GL value into the table above we can begin to see the significance of the GL rating system:

FOOD	GI Value	GL Value
Burgen mixed grain bread	34	2 slices = 4 GL
Muffin	54	11 GL
Special K cereal	54	30g = 14GL
Cola drink	63	250ml = 14GL
Croissant	67	1 = 17GL
Weetabix	69	2 biscuits = 11 GL
Wholemeal bread	69	1 thick slice = 9GL
Crumpet	69	1 = 13GL

Bagel	69	1 = 24GL
Swede	72	150g = 7GL
Watermelon	72	120g = 4GL
Gluten free bread	79	1 slice = 10GL
Cornflakes	84	30g = 21GL
Puffed wheat	89	30g = 16GL
Rice milk	92	250ml = 14GL

Under the GI rating system, Special K would be considered fine to eat, having a score of 54. But we can see that because it is all unrefined carbs it has a GL value of 14! Okay if you're wanting to maintain your weight, but not if you want to lose weight.

A bagel, just squeezes into the "eat in moderation" bracket yet has a massive GL value of 24! That blows 2 main meals and 1 snack in just 1 bagel!!!

Puffed wheat has a high GI score of 89 which is reflected in the GL value of 16. One meal and 1 snacks worth!

However, look more closely at watermelon with a GI value of 72 which puts it into the "avoidance" group. It has so little sugar (just 6 grams) in it that the GL value is only 4, making it fine to eat. If we do the math with watermelon we can see how this works out:

72 x 6 = 432 divided by 100 = 4.32   rounded to 4GL per serving.

When you start looking at the GL value of foods, it becomes evident how easy it is to blow your blood sugar levels and mess up your diet. Snacking on a 250ml can of cola with a crumpet is a massive GL value of 27! I've known many people who drink nothing but cola, having up to 2 litres a day and can't understand why they feel so ill.

Getting your diet back to basics is crucial if you want to avoid the disease conditions that are almost epidemic in the western world.

To summarise: Avoid all processed, packaged, "free from", low sugar, low fat and microwaveable foods. Use the recipes from my Eating to Get Pregnant book and prepare your meals using fresh, organic, free range produce. Think about how far your food has travelled and how it is prepared. Factory-processed food which uses cheap ingredients, sugar and flavouring, hydrogenated fats just isn't going to provide you with the nutrients you need to make a healthy baby.

Finally, don't <u>ever</u> microwave anything that goes in your mouth. Your food may come out of the microwave looking the same as it did when it went in there only hotter, but remember that microwaves damage the molecular structure and destroy the nutrient content of food. The net result is that instead of your body receiving the nourishment it needs, it is presented with a toxic product that it cannot digest and needs to get rid of as soon as possible.

EATING TO MAXIMISE FERTILITY.

Have lots of variety in your diet to make sure you get all the vitamins, minerals, fats and proteins you need. It's no good just eating carrots and peas with your Sunday dinner and expecting to have healthy sperm and eggs! (And some people do!)

Dump white bread, processed foods, biscuits, cakes, cookies, chips.

Instead, eat granary bread, fresh fruit and vegetables, whole grains such as porridge oats, nuts, seeds and good quality proteins.

Having some protein with each meal will slow down the rate at which the sugar content of carbs is released. Ideally, eat small amounts little and often and take time to enjoy your food and listen to your body when it tells you that it is satisfied by what you've eaten. (And then STOP).

Fruit And Vegetables

Make sure that you both include all of the following in your diet:-

At least 5 portions (preferably 7) of fruit and vegetables every day. Make sure they are lightly cooked or raw to preserve the vitamin, mineral and fibre content.

In order to alkalise your body, eat a salad each day and incorporate a wide range of different fruits and vegetables. Go for the "rainbow effect" on your plate. Regularly eating fruit and vegetables can halve your risk of miscarriage.

Complex Carbohydrates

Eat complex carbohydrates as they are your key source of energy and vital fertility boosting nutrients such as zinc, selenium and B vitamins. Complex carbohydrates are found in vegetables, wholemeal bread, oats, wholemeal pasta, brown rice, pulses and beans.

Avoid simple carbohydrates in the form of white bread, cakes, pastry, white flour, sugar which have little or no nutritional value and disrupt your blood sugar levels. Fruit is okay as it contains vital nutrients which are important for fertility.

Including whole grains, fruit and vegetables in your diet should ensure that you get plenty of fibre. Fibre is needed to keep your bowels healthy, clear out toxins and old hormone residues. Don't add bran to your food as it actually blocks the absorption of vital nutrients such as iron and zinc.

If you suffer from constipation, soak a tablespoon of organic linseeds (flaxseeds) overnight in water then add the whole lot to porridge or muesli in the morning.

Drink Water

Drink at least 6 glasses of water every day. Water is essential for hormone balance, transporting nutrients to your organs, removal of toxins and metabolising stored fat. Drink little and often through the day. Flavour water with fresh orange or lemon slices or try herb or fruit teas. If you drink tap water, filter it first.

Don't drink with a meal as you will dilute your digestive juices and make it more difficult for your system to digest and absorb what you eat.

Protein

Protein foods are needed for building and repairing cells, manufacturing hormones and a healthy reproductive system. You do not store proteins and so need a constant supply.

Try eating a small amount of good quality protein with every meal. Good sources of protein are oily fish such as salmon, trout, sardines; eggs; pulses; beans and beansprouts; nuts and seeds; meat and poultry.

Make sure that you have free range/organic meat and poultry. Factory reared chickens contain more fat than protein and should be avoided. If you have fibroids, endometriosis or PCOS then you are best to avoid red meats, otherwise keep it to a maximum of twice a week.

Avoid dairy foods if you can. Modern production methods mean that dairy cows are milked when they are pregnant and so high levels of oestrogen are present in the milk. This carries over into all dairy products which are known to increase oestrogen levels in the blood. Try having sheep, goats, Hemp or soya milk instead.

Essential Fatty Acids (EFAs)

Fat is an essential part of your diet and cutting all fat out will lead to a wide variety of serious health problems. However, fats can be divided into two groups; those that help your body to function and increase fertility and those that contribute to its destruction. The fats that you need are fresh, unprocessed fats containing one or both of the essential Omega 3 and Omega 6 fatty acids.

Omega 3 fatty acids are vital to the development of a baby's brain, eyes and nervous system. It is also needed for the maintenance and repair of your brain and nervous system. Omega 3s are anti-inflammatory and deficiency has been linked with a number of health ailments. Your body also relies on fats as an energy source.

Essential fatty acids are found in oily fish, avocadoes, nuts and seeds. People often avoid nuts, thinking that the high fat content will make them put on weight, but the essential fats that nuts contain actually help your body to metabolise stored fat.

As I said before, you need to avoid trans-fats and hydrogenated fats. These are the fats which have undergone chemical processing which changes their molecular structure, making them damaging to the body. This kind of fat is most commonly found in fried foods, cakes, biscuits, chips, pastries, margarine, processed foods, crisps and "fast food".

Eating 4g of trans-fats daily (the equivalent of half a portion of takeaway fried chicken) has been shown to cause problems with ovulation and reduce fertility. However, essential fatty acids can improve fertility for both men and women.

Studies have shown that children born to mothers who ate at least 350g of oily fish every week had more advanced motor, communication and social skills. The housewives tale that fish makes you clever is proving to be true, as it is now known to be vital to proper brain function throughout life.

Get Back To Basics and Include Some Superfoods

In the companion recipe book Eating to Get Pregnant, you'll find lots of ideas to help you plan your meals. The recipes are all designed to be alkalising and stay within the guidelines for 15GL for each meal.

I suggest that you try out some of the daily menus until you get the hang of planning your meals and snacks for the day, then dip in and out of the recipes. The key "ingredient" in all of the recipes is to use fresh foods which you prepare yourself.

I really encourage you to put thought into your meals, take time to think about the ingredients, try new ideas and remember that what you put in your mouth becomes you.

Cultivate Good Eating Habits

Stress is the most powerful anti-nutrient. If you are not in an optimum state of relaxation when you eat, it doesn't matter if you eat the most healthy, organic food, your body simply cannot absorb the nutrients within it.

Eating when your digestion is switched off means that:-

- Nutrient absorption goes down

- Calcium, magnesium, zinc, chromium and selenium are excreted through the urine
- Cholesterol levels go up
- Triglyceride levels go up
- Blood platelets go sticky
- Cortisol signals your body to store fat
- Good bacteria are killed off
- Growth hormone decreases
- Thyroid hormone decreases
- The risk of Osteoporosis goes up
- You are more likely to suffer bloating, cramps, indigestion.

Learn how to improve your metabolism through pleasure and relaxation!

One of your body's "pleasure" chemicals called Cholecystokinin is produced in response to protein and fats in a meal and has 3 interesting functions. (i) it stimulates the intestines to prepare for digestion, (ii) it shuts down digestion when you've had enough and (iii) it stimulates a pleasure sensation.

This same chemical that helps digest your meal also tells you when it's time to stop eating and makes you feel good about the whole experience! Pleasure, metabolism and a naturally controlled appetite are very closely linked. The more you enjoy your food the better your digestion!

When you are stressed and your SNS has released adrenaline, breathing tends to be more rapid, arrhythmic and shallow. Movement tends to be quicker than usual. Your brain associates shallow breathing and rapid movement with being stressed.

On the other hand, when your PNS is activated you are relaxed, breathing is relaxed, deep and rhythmic and movements are slower. Your brain knows that when you take deep, slow breaths you are usually relaxed, therefore you are not in danger.

You can use this information to fool your brain and get it to activate the PNS, thereby SWITCHING ON digestion whenever you eat.

Follow these golden rules:

When you relax your breathing, your whole body relaxes and digestion is optimised. Before every meal, take 5 deep breaths. Breathe in for a count of 5, hold for a count of 5 and breathe out for a count of 5. Pause whilst you are eating and take a deep breath and oxygenate your digestive system. Remember, your body needs oxygen for efficient fuel (food) burning.

Eat slowly - remember that even though you may feel happy and relaxed, if you eat quickly, you will switch on the stress response.

Give yourself time to eat. Sit down, play some quiet relaxing music, <u>enjoy your food.</u>

Make eating a time when you give to yourself. Give yourself space, <u>enjoy your food.</u>

If you are anxious, ask yourself if the situation is life threatening. If not, allow yourself to relax through breathing.

Turn off the television, put the newspaper aside and don't answer the phone when eating.

Don't multi-task when eating. Don't read your emails, work, or look at your computer. As soon as you do this, your brain is thrown into a state of confusion and stress because it doesn't know where you want it to pay attention. Remember stress switches off digestion.

Include As Many Of These "Superfoods" In Your Diet As You Possibly Can:-

Sprouted beans and seeds

These are newly germinated seeds and pulses, baby plants bursting with all of the concentrated nutrition necessary to produce a fully grown plant.

Sprouts are a powerhouse of nutrients.

- All the trace minerals including selenium and zinc.
- Antioxidant nutrients such as Vitamins A, C, B and E.
- Bioflavonoids
- Amino acids (the building blocks of protein)
- Antioxidant enzymes.
- Fibre
- RNA and DNA which are anti-ageing.
- Protein
- Calcium

Eating sprouts regularly can result in an enormous improvement in your general health, boosting the immune system, revitalising and strengthening the body, improving digestion, combating tiredness and stress.

Sprouted beans and seeds can be added to salads, stir fries, soups, casseroles or eaten on their own. If you are adding them to cooked food, add them for no more than 1 minute at the end just to warm them through. If you cook sprouts to a high temperature you will simply destroy all of the wonderful nutrients they contain.

Beansprouts are an important source of protein for vegetarians and vegans and are soooo cheap!

Pomegranite Seeds

Like all red fruits, pomegranite is rich in antioxidants. One glass of pomegranate juice contains an entire day's supply of folic acid, perfect for helping conceive healthy babies.

Drinking pure pomegranate juice has been shown to help stabilize blood sugar levels, another cause of infertility and PCOS. When buying pomegranite juice check the label for added sugar, in particular look for high fructose corn syrup (HFCS).

Pomegranite seeds are delicious and go well with green salads or added to desserts.

Chia Seeds

Chia, seeds have more omega-3 fatty acids than salmon, a wealth of antioxidants and minerals, a complete source of protein and more fibre than flax seed. They can help regulate blood sugar levels and because they are also very high in zinc, they are great for male fertility.

Blended into a smoothie, their mild flavor vanishes. Chia seeds are tasteless cooked with hot cereal and are great stirred into porridge.

Hemp Seeds

Hemp seeds contain all the essential amino acids and essential fatty acids necessary to maintain healthy human life. No other single plant source has the essential amino acids in such an easily digestible form, nor has the essential fatty acids in as perfect a ratio to meet human nutritional needs.

Hemp seed is a nutritious dietary source of easily digestible gluten-free protein. It provides a well-balanced array of all the amino acids, including 34.6g of protein per 100g. The fatty acid profile of the hemp seed is extremely beneficial, containing omega-6 and omega-3 fatty acids in a virtually ideal ratio.

Other beneficial aspects of hemp seed include a strongly favourable ratio of unsaturated/saturated fat; a high content of antioxidants; and a wide variety of vitamins and minerals.

Shelled hemp seeds are delicious when added to salads or to a breakfast muesli.

Avocados

Avocados are rich, creamy, and filling. Although they're often shunned for being "fattening" (they average about 300 calories each, mostly from fat), avocados are actually heart-healthy if you eat them in moderation.

Their oils are mostly monounsaturated - the kind that lowers LDL ("bad") cholesterol but maintains HDL ("good") cholesterol. Many people think avocados have cholesterol, but no plant foods do.

Avocados provide important nutrients, including folate, vitamins C and E, and potassium, as well as fibre (about 12g in each). Their phytochemicals include beta-sitosterol (a natural sterol that lowers cholesterol), glutathione (an antioxidant that may protect against certain cancers), and lutein (a carotenoid that may help protect against macular degeneration and cataracts). Recent research from Ohio State University showed that avocados can significantly boost absorption of carotenoids from other foods, suggesting you should add a bit of avocado to your salads in place of less-healthful toppings. They are also delicious when whizzed into a vegetable/fruit juice (see below).

Coconut

Coconut is highly nutritious and rich in fibre, vitamins, and minerals. It is classified as a "functional food" because it provides many health benefits beyond its nutritional content.

The flesh of coconut contains Vitamin C, Thiamin, Riboflavin, Niacin, Pantothenic acid, Vitamin B-6, Folate, Vitamin B-12, Vitamin A, Retinol, Vitamin E (alpha-tocopherol), Vitamin K, a range of minerals including calcium, selenium and magnesium AND amino acids. A true superfood!

Use coconut oil for cooking in place of saturated oils. Use coconut milk to make a satisfying smoothie by adding a banana and raw egg. Eat coconut flesh as a snack food.

Green Supplements

Green plants contain chlorophyll which is the result of sunlight being converted into energy during the process of photosynthesis. Green powder supplements are nutrient rich and include easily digested protein.

One of the best green powders I've found is Juicemasters Ultimate Superfoods (available from www.juicemaster.com). It contains Barley Grass, Wheat Grass, Nettle Leaf, Shavegrass (Horsetail), Alfalfa Leaf Juice, Dandelion Leaf Juice, Kamut® Grass Juice, Barley Grass Juice, Oat Grass Juice, Burdock Root, Broccoli Juice, Kale Juice, Spinach Juice, Parsley Juice, Carob Pod, Ginger Root, Nopal Cactus, Alma Berry, Spirulina and Chlorella.

It's great when added to a juice or water and as well as delivering a powerhouse of nutrients it helps to alkalise your blood and tissues.

Juicing

Juicing is a great way to get lots of vital nutrients into your body in a way that is easily absorbed. Having a freshly made juice each day can give you loads of energy, keep blood sugar levels stable and help you lose any excess weight. (Getting down to your ideal weight is really important, as excess fat stores have a negative influence on hormones for both men and women.)

You can add avocado, Green Powder or bee pollen to a juice to make it even more nutrient dense. There's so much to say in favour of juicing that I strongly recommend you read any book on juicing by Jason Vale.

You'll find some of my favourite juice recipes for fertility in the companion recipe book.

Jason Vales website is www.juicemaster.com where you can buy his books and juicers.

Bee Pollen: Bee Pollen contains nearly all the nutrients required by humans, all the essential amino acids, a full spectrum of vitamins and minerals, trace elements, enzymes (including anti-oxidants), and hormone precursors which stimulate hormone production and help anti-aging. About half of its protein is in the form of free amino acids that are ready to be used directly by the body. Such highly assimilable protein can contribute significantly to your protein needs.

Bee pollen can be taken as grains straight off the spoon, added to breakfast cereal or added to a smoothie or vegetable juice.

Bee Pollen can be taken in tablet form if you prefer, I would recommend Solgar as a reliable make.

The Vital Nutrients For Fertility

Beta Carotene Your body turns beta carotene into Vitamin A and good levels are needed before conception takes place as it's essential to the developing embryo. It's best not to have high doses of Vitamin A from animal sources such as liver as this can cause birth defects.

Found in: safe vegetable sources - tomatoes, green plants, mangoes, pumpkin, cabbage, egg yolk, parsley, broccoli, carrots, sweet potatoes, apricots, squash, red and green peppers

Vitamin B6 can more than double your chances of getting pregnant. It's needed for making female sex hormones and regulating oestrogen and progesterone levels.

Women who have plenty of B6 in their diet halve their chances of miscarriage in the early weeks, possibly because B6 plays an important role in the development of the placenta.

Found in: Potatoes, whole grains, chickpeas, mushrooms, oats, soya beans, seaweeds, sunflower seeds, salmon, mackerel, raisins, lentils, bananas, avocado, cabbage, molasses, eggs, milk products

Vitamin B12 is essential for the health of your nervous system, production of red blood cells and fertility.

Found in: Sardines, seaweed, trout, salmon, lamb, eggs, lean beef, edam cheese, cottage cheese

Folic Acid is an important B vitamin known mainly for its role in preventing spina bifida and should be supplemented in the pre-conception period. It also plays an important role in fertility.

Found in: blackeye peas, green beans, broccoli, green peas, salmon, alfalfa sprouts, chick peas, oranges, strawberries, wholemeal bread, beans & pulses, lentils, green leafy vegetables, asparagus, oatmeal, dried figs, avocado

Vitamin C has been shown to help trigger ovulation and increase sperm count by up to a third. Also helps to prevent sperm clumping together.

Found in: raw fruits and vegetables, citrus fruits, blueberries, red peppers, kale, parsley, watercress, broccoli, kiwi fruit, strawberries, blackcurrants, papaya, spinach, oranges, cabbage, melon, mango, lemon

Vitamin E helps with sperm and hormone function and is associated with a reduced risk of miscarriage.

Found in: whole grains, whole grains, egg yolk, green leafy vegetables, lettuce, nuts, sesame seeds, organic cold pressed nut & seed oils (sesame, walnut), avocado, oily fish, broccoli

Calcium Essential not just for the health of bones and teeth in both mother and child but also the nervous system and blood.

Found in: sardines, salmon, prunes, almonds, oranges, papaya, watermelon, nuts, whole grains, parsley, watercress, spinach, broccoli, cottage cheese, sesame seeds, linseeds, tofu, yoghurt, bony fish, figs, kelp, molasses, hard cheese (edam, gouda),

Selenium deficiency has been linked to an increased risk of miscarriage.

Found in: eggs, avocado, carrots, mushroom, broccoli, brazil nuts, garlic, butter, barley, smoked herring, brown rice, wheat germ, oats, wholegrains, red swiss chard

Zinc deficiency in women can lead to reduced fertility and increase risk of miscarriage. It is needed for the production of sperm and male hormones and the development of the unborn baby.

Found in: eggs, apricots, dried fruits, seaweed, watermelons, mushrooms, beetroot, oily fish, onions, lean meat, fish, chicken, eggs, pumpkin seeds, sunflower seeds, whole grains, legumes, ginger root, split peas, rye, oats, parsley

Manganese deficiency has been linked to behavioural problems in children and an increased risk of a child being born with a physical malformation. It's needed for healthy skin, bone and cartilage formation and to regulate blood sugar levels.

Found in: pecans, whole grains, seeds, sweet potatoes, onions, green beans, parsley, strawberries, apples, spinach, brazil nuts, barley, oats, rye, raisins, buckwheat, turnip greens, split peas, beet greens, walnuts, brussels sprouts, cornmeal, millet, carrots, broccoli, brown rice, green leafy vegetables, ginger, eggs, parsley, thyme

Magnesium is necessary as an anti-stress mineral, keeping the circulatory system healthy. It counterbalances calcium and is an important fertility mineral affecting a woman's ability to conceive and sustain a pregnancy.

Found in: almonds, nuts, eggs, avocado, sunflower seeds, kelp, green leafy vegetables, tofu, legumes, rye, buckwheat, millet, molasses, brown rice, bananas, dried figs, dried apricots, barley

Chromium is essential for proper utilisation of carbohydrates and stabilizes blood sugar. This is an important mineral for anyone struggling to control their blood sugar level. It is particularly relevant to anyone with PCOS.

Found in: wheat germ, rye bread, potatoes, green pepper, apples, butter, parsnips, cornmeal, banana, spinach, carrots, blueberries, green beans, butter, cabbage, oysters, clams, yeast, egg yolk, cheese, molasses

Iron is essential for making red blood cells which transport oxygen round the body, it's necessary for energy and vitality. It has been shown to help women improve their fertility.

Found in: meat (lean), sardines, chicken, eggs, kelp, molasses, pumpkin seeds, broccoli, oatmeal, spinach, parsley, dried apricots, dried figs, dried peaches, prunes, Spirulina, seafood, dried yeast, wholemeal bread,

Potassium works to control the activity of heart muscles, nervous systems and kidney, keeps tissues in good tone.

Found in: bananas, avocado, carrots, pineapple, leafy green vegetables, lima beans, potato, tomato, apples, dried apricots, peaches,
Melon, wheat bran, dried fruit, nuts, muesli, vegetables, soya beans, red peppers

Do you see how simple foods such as vegetables,

nuts, seeds, beans and lentils provide a wide spectrum of the essential vitamins and minerals for fertility?

You'll find some delicious recipes in the companion recipe book "Eating to Get Pregnant".

FACTORS AFFECTING SPERM HEALTH

The testes are outside the male body because they need to be kept cooler than body temperature. It's important for the man to wear loose clothing, cotton underpants and to avoid hot saunas or baths. Compression of the testes due to cycling, sitting all day or having thick thighs can all affect sperm health.

Cyclists can buy saddles with indents to accommodate the testes, taxi or lorry drivers can try sitting on a ring such as a child's swimming ring. If you use a laptop don't sit it on your lap to use it, place it on a desk and don't keep a mobile phone in your trouser pocket.

Sperm are particularly vulnerable to what is known as oxidative stress or free radical damage. Free radicals are unstable molecules that are linked with cellular destruction and high levels endanger sperm function and viability.

 Some causes are poor nutrition, pollutants such as smoking and poor detoxification processes by the body. Burnt, fried and barbequed foods are also sources of free radicals. Damage often results in abnormally formed sperm, and a poor morphology result. Free radicals can also cause sperm to become hyperactive whilst still in the reproductive tract which affects their motility.

Semen normally contains agents known as anti-oxidants to protect sperm against free radicals and if in some way this natural defence system is impaired, the effect on sperm can be extremely damaging. Therefore it is essential to both remove potential causes of free radical damage and to eat a diet high in anti-oxidants.

Sources of free radicals

Smoking

Processed foods, particularly foods high in artificial additives

Fast foods

Alcohol

Recreational drugs

Foods that contain high amounts of poor quality fats and oils, particularly processed meats, margarines, biscuits and pastries, and take-aways.

Fried, BBQd and burnt foods

Exposure to environmental pollution such as traffic fumes. Keep car windows closed in traffic jams and wear a mask if you cycle.

The most potent anti-oxidants for improving male fertility are:

Vitamin E: This is a fat-soluble vitamin and the main anti-oxidant in sperm membranes. It works with selenium in its anti-oxidative capacity. If you are taking prescribed medicines for blood pressure or blood thinning medications such as aspirin, heparin or warfarin please seek advice from your Doctor before taking vitamin E.

Selenium: This antioxidant mineral is vital for healthy sperm formation, particularly motility. It also protects against toxic metal contamination. Consumption of selenium in food is dependent on the amount in the soil where the food is grown, and it is believed that the soil is often highly depleted of this mineral, so supervised supplementation is especially recommended.

Ascorbic Acid (Vitamin C): Vitamin C is a water-soluble vitamin and its most important role in male fertility is the prevention of agglutination, when sperm clump together. This often happens when anti-bodies bind to sperm and can be a result of present or past genito-urinary infection. Vitamin C is also a powerful anti-oxidant and present in high levels in seminal fluid. Over- heating and smoking easily destroy it.

Other Important Nutrients In Male Fertility:

Zinc: Zinc is a trace mineral, and perhaps one of the most well known nutrients important in male fertility.

Zinc deficiency decreases both testosterone and sperm counts. It is highly concentrated in the seminal fluid and seminal plasma zinc concentration is significantly correlated with sperm density, motility and viability. However zinc supplementation needs to be carefully monitored because too high doses can impair immune function.

L-Arginine: This is an amino acid that may affect both sperm count and motility. The heads of sperm contain large amounts and abnormal sperm counts often indicate a deficiency of arginine in the semen.

Note: People who suffer from the herpes virus should avoid foods rich in arginine as it stimulates the virus to replicate.

Foods rich in Arginine are nuts especially walnuts, almonds, brazil nuts, beans, lentils

L-Carnitine: This amino acid plays a crucial role in the metabolic processes of energy production that fuel sperm motility and high levels are normally found in sperm cells. Vegetarians should be aware that there is virtually no carnitine in plant foods, and supplementation can be important

Foods rich in Carnitine are beef, pork, lamb, dairy products

Co-enzyme Q10: Co-enzyme Q10 is a vital catalyst in the conversion of food to energy within cells. In sperm cells it is concentrated in the mid piece where it is an energy promoter and anti-oxidant. Research is showing that it may be effective in improving fertilisation rates following ICSI. It can help improve sperm motility

In addition, vitamins B12 and folic acid, the amino acid taurine and the anti-oxidant glutathione are all important for fertility. Vitamins C and E, zinc, selenium, Co-enzyme Q10, Carnitine and Arginine are all vital to sperm health.

SUPPLEMENTING YOUR DIET

Research from the University of Leeds shows that taking a good quality multi-vitamin and mineral can double your chances of getting pregnant.

There are a number of good quality fertility supplements available and I recommend these:

Fertility Plus for women and Fertility Plus for men, as used by Dr Marilyn Glenville. Available from www.naturalhealthpractice.com

Zita West Vitafem for Women and Vitamen for men. Available from www.zitawest.com

If you want to use an over the counter fertility supplement, it's worth checking the ingredient list against the list below to make sure you're getting all that you need.

You both need:

Folic Acid   400ug
Zinc   30mg
Selenium   100ug
Vitamin B6   20mg
Vitamin B5   20mg
Biramin B1   20mg
Vitamin B12   20ug
Vitamin E   160mg

Vitamin C   1000mg
Vitamin d   2.5ug
Beta
Carotene   up to 5mg
Chromium   20ug

He also needs:

L- arginine   300mg
L – carnitine 100mg

Omega 3 Essential fatty acids:

Changes in our eating patterns over the last century has resulted in eight out of ten women being deficient in docosahexaenoic acid (DHA).   Omega 3 fats are important for regulating reproductive hormones and supporting the development of the babys brain, eyes and central nervous system.

Prostaglandins are produced from essential fatty acids and these have hormone like functions.   In women they help prevent low birth weight and premature birth.   It helps to prevent blood from clotting inappropriately and so may be helpful where there is a history of miscarriage linked to a clotting problem.

In men, semen should be rich in prostaglandins and low levels can lead to sperm abnormalities.

I recommend taking Fish Oil capsules which are rich in the fatty acids you need. 1000mg daily. Don't take Cod Liver Oil capsules, these are produced from the cod's liver which can contain high levels of toxins. They contain high levels of vitamin A, which is not recommended in this form in pregnancy.

If you prefer not to take a fish oil capsule, you should instead take a linseed oil capsule. The body has to convert linseed oil into essential fatty acids so it is a less efficient way to get these vital nutrients.

Folic acid:

If you choose not to take extra supplements, just make sure you are getting enough folic acid in your everyday diet as the research clearly shows that this prevents neural tube defects, such as spina bifida. Women with chronic conditions such as epilepsy or diabetes may require a higher dose of folic acid, so speak to your GP.

Minimizing The Risk Of Miscarriage

There are many factors that can cause a miscarriage. Some may not be in your control, but some certainly are. Everything that you eat or drink, even inhale enters your bloodstream and crosses the placenta to your baby. In the early stages of pregnancy, the baby's organs are still underdeveloped and they can't cope with toxins which can harm them.

If the toxic load is too great and causes too much damage, the baby will not continue to develop as it should, leading to miscarriage.

I've already talked about some of the toxins which you need to avoid to create the healthiest eggs and sperm. But let's look at the factors regarding miscarriage.

Miscarriage is most likely to happen in the first trimester.

Caffeine

Research shows that 200mg of caffeine a day increases the risk of miscarriage. That's as little as 2 cups of coffee a day. Women who drink more than 200 mg of caffeine a day have double the risk of miscarriage, with a 25 % higher risk compared to a 12 % risk of a miscarriage in women who didn't consume caffeine. Remember that caffeine is also present in green tea, black tea, cola drinks and some energy drinks.

There are plenty of alternative drinks which you can find in a good health store. If you feel you must have coffee, limit yourself to one cup of decaffeinated coffee. Look for a brand that has been water decaffeinated as chemical decaffeination processes simply switch the caffeine for a toxic chemical.

Smoking

Reasearch shows that smoking in pregnancy is one of the most common causes of miscarriage, stillbirth, premature delivery and low birth weight. Various researchers suggest that the babys IQ can be reduced between 6 and 15 points if the mother smokes.

Miscarriages more commonly occur when the male partner has low sperm counts and abnormal sperm. Smoking severely impacts the quality and quantity of sperm. Scientists have discovered that when men quit smoking for 5-15 months sperm count is increased by 50- 800% on average respectively.

Mercury

Mercury is known to cause neurological problems in the developing baby, as well as other development problems. The United States Environmental Protection Agency (US EPA) have already issued preventative warnings to pregnant or nursing women to avoid including seafood in their diet because of the possibility of heavy metal contamination.

Tuna, king mackerel, sushi and sashimi all have high levels of mercury and should be avoided.

Electromagnetic (EM) radiation

Diagnostic or therapeutic radiotherapy, X-rays are potentially harmful to your baby. If you are pregnant or trying to get pregnant discuss this with your doctor before being exposed to any form of electromagnetic radiation.

Also bear in mind that EM radiation emitted from computers, mobile phones and wireless networks at home can be another one of the things that cause miscarriage.

Alcohol

Regular alcohol consumption during pregnancy can cause miscarriages. Heavy drinking or binge drinking can cause stillbirth as well as other developmental problems in the fetus. Also, your baby might acquire a disorder know as fetal alcohol syndrome. It's recommended you stop drinking alcohol both during pregnancy and for at least 3 months before trying to get pregnant.

Drugs

A study by Canadian researchers report found that antidepressant drugs taken during pregnancy may increase the likelihood of miscarriage by 68%. In the study of over 5, 000 pregnant women, those taking antidepressants called selective serotonin reuptake inhibitors (SSRIs) had a higher risk of miscarriage.

Aspartame

We've already discussed aspartame and how it changes to formaldehyde, but it's worth noting that It may even turn to formic acid, a far more toxic compound than formaldehyde. Formaldehyde in the mother's blood stream can cause her immune system to see the fetal tissue as foreign substance and so attack and kill it.

Zinc deficiency

Zinc is needed to properly maintain pregnancy in women and produce healthy sperm in men. Artificial hormones in the form of oral contraceptives and ovulation drugs can significantly reduce its levels.
Zinc helps to regulate androgens and lower levels of prolactin. This function helps prevent PCOS, infertility, hair loss.

Zinc is critical to the production of testosterone, and the production and motility of sperm. (Remember healthy sperm are needed to prevent miscarriage.)

Some symptoms of zinc deficiency are:

- Frequent colds and infections
- White spots on fingernails
- Mental exhaustion
- Poor appetite
- Dry skin and hair
- Poor sense of taste and smell

Boost your zinc levels by including in your diet lean beef, whole grains, eggs, peas, nuts, pumpkin seeds, poultry, clams and oysters.

Progesterone Deficiency

Progesterone is needed to maintain the pregnancy. Progesterone deficiency may lead to PMS and short menstrual cycles.

Ensure you have adequate intake of magnesium and vitamin B6 for production of progesterone.
Foods like seeds, nuts and egg yolk are rich in B vitamins and dark green leafy vegetables, whilst legumes and nuts are a good source of magnesium.

Vitamin C deficiency

The strength of the lining of your uterus (womb) is crucial when you are trying to conceive and stay pregnant. More commonly than not, when the connective tissue is weak the embryo will not be able to attach or stay attached.

The quality of the connective tissue and blood vessels depends on how much vitamin C and bioflavonoids are present in the body. Bioflavonoids help the body absorb more vitamin C and also contribute to the strength of the connective tissue.

Boost your Vitamin C intake by eating lemons, limes, grapefruit, kiwi, berries, peppers, broccoli and guava.

ASSISTED CONCEPTION

Many of the couples that I see for fertility find to their delighted surprise that once they put into place all the guidelines in Part One, they conceive naturally.

However, year on year I see an increasing number of couples who need assisted conception and particularly couples who have no medical reason for not getting pregnant. The diagnosis "unexplained infertility" seems to apply to a high percentage of couples.

This can be an emotional and stressful time. On the one hand you're disappointed that you haven't got pregnant naturally, but on the other hand you feel like you're taking control and being pro-active.

It's ironic that for many women they are in control of their fertility when they take the contraceptive pill, yet when they decide they want to get pregnant nothing happens.

Your first port of call will be your doctor. You should tell your doctor how long you've been trying to conceive and ask for a referral to your local fertility clinic or specialist. When they've done all the necessary tests, you may then be offered treatment.

I always suggest to a couple that they should have a conversation *before* they embark on any assisted conception programme. This conversation needs to cover:

- how important having a child is to *both* of them?
- what they are each willing to do to improve their fertility?
- how far they are willing to go to have a child i.e. what kind of fertility treatment will they have?
- how many treatments will they consider?
- when will they know it's time to stop?

I think it's best to have this conversation before embarking on any assisted conception programme. I've seen so many cases where the first 2 or 3 IVF protocols failed and the woman is thinking "next time it'll work – next time I'll have acupuncture and that will make it work." It's emotionally draining for both partners and physically exhausting for the woman. That's without factoring in the financial cost.

I've seen women who were willing to travel abroad and use both donor sperm and eggs even though they were so exhausted physically and emotionally, they were in no fit state to get pregnant.

It's so difficult when your body clock is ticking and every period reminds you of your inability to get pregnant, to make the best long-term decisions. These are decisions that you must make together, and, you must feel that should you decide to go ahead with assisted conception you're both 100% committed to the process.

Do spend time researching your options before you go ahead with fertility treatment.   Your local clinic may be convenient, but does it have a good track record?   Can you speak to other patients and ask them about their experiences?   Does the clinic have an open evening you can both go to?

Check that the clinic offers a 7 day a week service. I've known of clinics who have a Monday to Friday service and they routinely use drugs such as norethisterone, to suppress a womans period so that it starts "on the right day of the week."   Egg collections and transfers are done on specific days and the woman must fit in with the clinics schedule.

Personally, I'm against giving a woman any more drugs than are strictly necessary.   Every woman responds differently to the treatment and I much prefer clinics who collect eggs and transfer embryos at the time that's right for the individual.

If you're in the UK, does the clinic offer any treatment under the N.H.S.? If so, what is on offer?

Ask about the clinics success rates for the procedure on offer. What is their cancellation rate? Sometimes a clinic will cancel a treatment protocol if it's not going well. That happens from time to time and is done in the best interests of the patient.

However a clinic may switch the status of an IVF treatment calling it a "trial stimulation" or change it to an IUI, so it doesn't get recorded as a failed IVF. The HFEA (Human Fertilisation Embryo Authority) only monitors conception that takes place outside the womb, so do be cautious if a clinic has a low cancellation rate.

Depending on which procedure you opt for, how frequently will you need to go for scans/tests? How will you manage that if you have a job or other children?

Once you're happy with the clinic you've chosen, it's time to decide on which fertility treatment you will go for.

On average, assisted reproduction has a 20% success. Much depends on your age and therefore the age of your eggs, the reasons for not conceiving, the number and quality of your embryos, your weight and emotional status.

If you are stressed and anxious, particularly through your fertility treatment this can potentially sabotage the process. I've noticed amongst my patients a definite pattern, if they are more relaxed, the higher the chance of success. This is why I have recorded guided meditations for you to listen to before and during your fertility treatment.

FOLLICULAR TRACKING

If your periods are irregular, then it can be very difficult to guage when you're ovulating. Your clinic may offer to scan you at weekly intervals during your cycle to determine when ovulation is likely to happen. You would then aim to have sex at the appropriate time and conceive naturally.

OVULATION INDUCTION

Provided that you your fallopian tubes and partners sperm are normal, you may be offered treatment to kick-start ovulation and help you conceive naturally.

The drug used is clomiphene citrate (brand name Clomid or Serophene), which is taken on days 2 to 5 of your cycle.

Clomiphene is an anti-oestrogen drug that binds to the oestrogen receptors in the brain tricking the brain into thinking that there is no oestrogen in the blood. This prompts the pituitary gland to release more FSH and LH stimulating a follicle to mature an egg.

Many women experience side effects from this drug such as headaches, nausea, bloating, depression and fatigue. However, clomiphene does stimulate ovulation in around 80% of women who were not ovulating and around 50% will conceive in 3 months.

Clomiphene does affect cervical secretions and the lining of the uterus and it also increases the rate of miscarriage. It's not advised to take clomiphene for more than 6 months due to the risk of ovarian cancer later in life. Ideally, you should have a break after 3 months before resuming treatment.

IUI – Intra Uterine Insemination

If clomiphene alone hasn't worked, the next phase is usually IUI. With IUI you may still be given clomiphene and monitored closely to make sure that you are not producing too many follicles. Three to four follicles is ideal so as not to run the risk of a multiple pregnancy.

The idea with IUI is to introduce the sperm high into the womb at ovulation time. This is to shorten the distance the sperm have to travel in order to reach the eggs.

It's not suitable for anyone with blocked fallopian tubes, poor egg quality or a very poor sperm count. Success rates vary from clinic to clinic but are around 10% at best. It is less invasive than an IVF treatment and can be a good way to monitor your response to stimulation. Many clinics will do 3 IUI treatments before moving on to IVF.

PREPARING FOR IVF

Before moving on to IVF I think it's really important to sit back, take stock and make sure that you are fully prepared for this treatment. You need to be sure that you've done everything you can to prepare your body.

General Health and fitness

1. If you are having repeated cycles of treatment allow a break of a month or two between cycles to allow your ovaries to recover.
2. IVF stands a better chance of working if you're not overweight or seriously underweight. Make sure you've followed the diet guidance in this book.
3. Don't smoke and avoid smoky atmospheres, as cigarette smoke affects the lining of the womb.

4. Avoid aerobic exercise once you start your cycle. As your hormonal system shuts down to prepare for IVF, your body needs rest. Gentle exercise such as walking and yoga is fine.
5. Limit the amount of time spent sitting at a desk / computer as this restricts blood flow. Rest and have early nights.

Reproductive Health

Ideally you will be having acupuncture in the lead up to starting your IVF cycle. Continue having weekly acupuncture from the time that you start your cycle up to egg collection. This will help to improve the flow of blood and energy to your reproductive organs, balance the body, build up the womb lining, grow follicles and help with implantation.

Keep your lower back and abdomen warm, particularly leading up to egg collection and between egg collection and transfer. Use a hot bag, hot water bottle or your hands. Do not use direct heat after embryo transfer.

Psychological and emotional preparation

Visualisation is very important at every stage of IVF. There are so many hurdles to overcome. Try not to allow yourself to slip into anxiety or negative thinking. At each stage of treatment, listen to the appropriate guided relaxation every day.

Explore other relaxation techniques to find one that suits you and fits into your life easily. Try yoga or tai chi.

Stress Management

IVF is potentially a stressful business so take time out occasionally to stop thinking and worrying and spend time with your partner doing things you both enjoy.

You need to be able to support each other through this and to still have a good relationship at the end of it. You'll both react differently to the pressures, so try to find ten minutes each evening to talk about what has happened and how you are feeling, so everything is out in the open.

Do not underestimate the time involved or the space you need to make in order to have IVF.

The guided relaxations are an excellent way to combat stress during the IVF process. Good breathing technique also helps to circulate oxygen around the body and into the reproductive organs.

THE IVF PROTOCOLS

The Long Protocol starts around day 21 of your cycle. You'll be given drugs to suppress or down-regulate your own hormones and stop any follicles developing. These drugs will usually be continued through the stimulation phase of your treatment to give the clinic complete control over when the follicles ripen and to minimise the risk of OHSS (Ovarian Hyperstimulation Syndrome).

The most commonly used down reg drugs are buserelin, nafarelin (synarel). With a day 21 start, you will have a period and then a baseline scan before you start to stimulate. The baseline scan is done to check that the ovaries are inactive and the lining of the womb is thin.

Down reg drugs put you into a temporary state of menopause. Some women experience hot flushes, headaches, mood changes and night sweats.

The stimulation phase will involve injections once or twice daily starting from day 3 of your cycle. The most commonly used drugs are Menopure, Menogon, Puragon, Gonal-F. Each of these drugs has a slightly different combination of FSH and LH and your clinic will decide which is the best for you. This is when it can be helpful to see how you have responded to IUI treatments.

You'll be scanned to monitor the progression of the follicles and the lining of your womb. Follicles should increase around 2ml a day and you want them to be around 18ml before the HCG injection and the lining of the womb to be around 8ml.   Once there are sufficient follicles of the right size you'll inject HcG, which simulates your natural LH surge, to bring the eggs to maturity ready for collection about 36 hours later.

Generally the clinic will aim to collect between 10 and 20 eggs.   But do remember that quality is more important than quantity. I've had patients who had 20 eggs collected, only half fertilised and the treatment failed. I've also had many more patients who have 8 to 10 eggs collected, most of them fertilise and they go on to get pregnant.

Egg collection is through the vaginal wall into the ovary, with one needle insertion per egg collected. This can create inflammation so it's important to rest and let your body heal after collection.

Once retrieved, the eggs will be put into a petri dish with the washed sperm sample and the embryologist will check them at intervals over the next day to see how many have fertilised and how well they are progressing.   The clinic will usually keep you informed of their progress.

Once cell division starts to happen, the embryologist will use his/her experience to advise on whether you should go for a 2 day transfer or wait till the embryos reach blastocyst stage, around 5 days after fertilisation. 2 to 3 day embryos will be put back into the womb on the assumption that this is the best place for them to continue to develop. Depending on quality, up to 2 embryos may be transferred.

If the embryos are developing well, they may be taken on to blastocyst stage when it will have around 120 cells. A blastocyst has a thin outer layer which develops into the placenta and they have cilia, tiny hairlike structures, which help them implant.

If an embryo reaches blastocyst stage it has about a 50% chance of implanting, and the embryologist will be able to select the embryo(s) which have progressed well. For many couples, the decision is made that they are better to go for a day 2 transfer. You can never know if an embryo that fails to develop to blastocyst in a petri dish, might have progressed if it had been returned to it's natural environment in the womb.

You really have to be confident in and trust the judgement of your embryologist to decide how best to proceed. When the embryos have been replaced in your womb you'll take progesterone to increase the chances of implantation.

If your hormonal cycle is not stable or regular, then the clinic may advise that the short protocol will be better for you. This is where the down regulation phase is skipped and you go straight to stimulation.

ICSI – INTRACYTOPLASMIC SPERM INJECTION

If the sperm are of poor quality or they can't penetrate the egg on their own, your clinic may recommend ICSI. ICSI might need to be used when there are no sperm in the semen sample and they have to be surgically retrieved.

In normal circumstances, the fittest, healthiest sperm will impregnate the egg. However, with ICSI a whole single sperm is injected into the egg with no way of knowing if it is the healthiest or fittest. There are concerns about ICSI increasing the risk of babies being born with chromosome defects. About 5% of injected eggs may be damaged by the ICSI process.

SUPPORTING THE PROCESS

The long protocol – down regulation/suppression

It's not easy to take a whole month off work, but be aware of what's happening to your hormonal system and slow down. Take things as easy as you possibly can and RELAX. Get plenty of early nights - sleep is very important for your body at this stage.

Allow plenty of time in your schedule for appointments - at least seven hours a week, depending on how often your clinic performs scans and blood tests and how long you're kept waiting at the clinic.

Use the appropriate guided relaxation for each phase every day. Tell yourself everything is working as it should be and that you are strong and healthy.

Get your partner involved in the process. It's so easy to leave them out until the time when they are called upon to give their semen sample. This can make them feel left out and create resentment on both sides.

Consider getting your partner to take charge of the drugs, making up the injections and telling you when you need to do them. If you're both comfortable with the idea, get your partner to do your injections for you.

161

Practise "injections" before you have to do the real thing. When I was training as an acupuncturist we had to do some practice needling on oranges before being let loose on a human body. Just get yourself a thick sewing needle and practise inserting it into an orange.

You'll find the skin quite thick and resistant and it's very similar to needling into a leg or stomach muscle. Keep your hand relaxed and imagine that you're pushing the needle right the way through the orange and out the other side. I've had a lot of patients practise this technique and they've found it much easier to do the injections.

Tips for the short protocol – stimulation phase

Stay relaxed and take each day as it comes. Anxiety and stress releases adrenaline into your blood stream. Spend some time each day sitting quietly and breathing deeply. Banish negative thoughts as they arise.

Repeat positive affirmations out loud: 'my eggs are growing, ripening and maturing; my eggs are of good quality; my womb lining is growing thick'. Imagine sending oxygen to your womb lining, helping it to grow. Visualise your eggs growing. Focus on how you want your body to respond.

Make sure that you drink plenty of water (at least 3 pints daily) and eat warm, nourishing foods. Have a little protein with each meal and snack.

Listen to the guided relaxations daily.

Egg collection and Transfer

Keep the lower abdomen warm up to and before egg collection. Do not use extra heat afterwards, just eat warm nourishing foods and keep warm.

A recent study has shown that women who had acupuncture before and after embryo transfer had a 42% success rate per cycle compared to 26% amongst those who did not. Studies also support the contribution that relaxation can make to improving conception rates.

Rest as much as you can and get plenty of early nights. After transfer, I recommend rest for a minimum of two to three days to give your embryos every possible chance to implant. You don't have to stay in bed, but just take things steady.

Don't feel guilty about taking time off and staying in bed if you wish. A gentle walk each day is fine.

The kidneys play an important role in reproduction according to Chinese medicine. They are especially active between 5pm and 7pm so this is a crucial time to rest quietly and a good time to listen to a relaxation.

AVOID caffeine, smoking, alcohol, sex, drugs, flying, heavy lifting, strenuous exercise, housework (including vacuuming), horse riding and aerobics, sun bathing, saunas, hot tubs, Jacuzzis, swimming and hot baths. Take a shower instead.

Make sure you listen to the appropriate guided relaxation every day. You'll find that they will help keep you calm and focussed. I always talk to my patients about their embryos still being connected to them on an energetic level.

They may physically be in a petri dish in an incubator, but they still have a connection with you. I really believe it's important to "talk" to your embryo(s) with your thoughts and let them know that they are being looked after and that you are looking forward to them returning to you.

Imagine that your embryo(s) are being cradled in warm, loving hands and surrounded by healing light. Remember, this is a stressful time for them too! You, at least, know what is going on but they have been plucked from their natural environment to be fertilised and grown. The guided relaxation will help you visualise this and I think it's important for you to feel that you're doing something for your embryo(s).

Continue to eat well, and have plenty of fluids.

The Two Week Wait

Make sure that you communicate with your partner. When you've had embryo transfer and you're in the 2 week wait you're on high alert for any signs that either the treatment has worked or failed.

Every twinge, breast tenderness, slight show will be analysed for its meaning and it's so easy to get yourself into a highly stressed and anxious state.

It's normal to have twinges, they can be implantation. Even period type pains are normal. The progesterone pessaries may cause breast tenderness. As far as you possibly can, find things to do to distract your mind. Read books or watch films you've been meaning to watch. Make time with your partner to just relax and be together. Remember this is a difficult time for them too.

Maintain a positive frame of mind. Once a fertilised embryo has been replaced in your uterus, hold the intention that you are pregnant and your body is doing all that it needs to in order to sustain the embryo. Until you have evidence to the contrary, hold that belief and don't let any negative thoughts creep in. Remember that your body responds to what you think, so focus on what you want to happen, not what you don't want.

Keep listening to the relaxations.

ACUPUNCTURE AND IVF

Acupuncture can support you with both preparing for IVF and throughout your treatment cycle.

Specifically, it can help alleviate any side effects from the drug regime and support the work of the drugs in both the down regulation and stimulation phases of the treatment. Research shows that acupuncture given before and after embryo transfer substantially increases the success rate of IVF.

I'd suggest finding an acupuncturist who is experienced in treating patients with fertility problems. Acupuncture is useful to help regulate your cycle, alleviate the symptoms of PCOS and endometriosis. It can also be used to help improve sperm quality.

Acupuncture can also be very useful to reduce your stress levels thereby helping to regulate your stress/fertility hormones.

If you want to try acupuncture to help you conceive, do take time to meet the person you intend to work with before starting treatment. Ask them about their experience in working with fertility and make sure that you feel comfortable with them A good practitioner will be an invaluable support to you in the coming months.

THE GUIDED RELAXATIONS

Earlier in the book I talked about the role of stress hormones and fertility hormones. Stress hormones are always prioritised over other hormones simply because they are our "get of trouble fast" hormones. They come into play whenever your brain perceives that there is a threat to your wellbeing.

I've talked about the importance of your diet and it's equally important to get control over your stress. The release of stress hormones is under the control of your autonomic nervous system (ANS), which I like to remember as the *automatic* nervous system. It regulates many processes in the body such as breathing, heart rate, without you needing to consciously think about it.

The ANS has 2 sides, one side (the SNS) switches on the stress response and the other side (the PNS) acts a counterbalance. The 2 sides should work together to maintain a state of balance in the body.

When you're anxious about anything at all, the SNS side is active. It makes you breathe more rapidly, increases heart rate, switches off digestion and pumps blood into your muscles to prepare you for flight or fight.

The PNS does the opposite, slowing down breathing and heart rate, optimising digestion and keeping blood circulating throughout the body. This is hugely important when you need to eat well, digest well and provide your ovaries with the nutrients they need to mature eggs. The lining of your womb needs a rich supply of blood to prepare for an embryo to embed.

Whenever I'm treating a woman through her IVF cycle I make time to talk her through some guided relaxation and visualisation at every treatment session. I tailor each relaxation according to where they are in the treatment cycle.

Research shows that stress can compromise the effectiveness of IVF treatment and that meditation supports the process. I've had numerous instances of women who've come to me for treatment because they have been so stressed throughout their fertility treatment. Women often ask if there is anything else they can do to improve their chances of success.

We've worked together and I've given them relaxations to listen to at home. In every case they have felt more relaxed and calm and the majority have gone on to have successful IVF treatments.

I've now recorded relaxations to accompany this book and you should choose the one that is relevant to where you are in your fertility journey. I really believe that positive visualisation, reducing stress and promoting a deep relaxation are important elements, particularly just before and after transfer of the embryo.

Each track is designed to help calm your mind and relax your body. Remember that thoughts affect your emotions and how your body responds. If you're stressed, anxious and negative your body responds by producing stress hormones. When you practice relaxation techniques the relaxation response kicks in making you calm and relaxed. The more you practice the better you'll be able to cope with the stress.

Never listen to a relaxation when you're driving. Take 20 minutes every day to do nothing else, just put your feet up or lie down and relax.

Track 1 – Preparing to get pregnant. (for both of you to listen to)

Track 2 - The down regulation phase of an IVF/ICSI cycle.

Track 3 – The stimulation phase of an IUI/IVF/ICSI cycle.

Track 4 – Pre egg collection IVF/ICSI cycle.

Track 5 – Post egg collection IVF/ICSI cycle.

Track 6 – Pre embryo transfer IVF/ICSI cycle.

Track 7 – Post embryo transfer IVF/ICSI cycle.

Track 8 – Pre treatment for IUI.

Track 9 – Post treatment for IUI.

Track 10 – The 2 week wait.

Track 11 – One for the men, visualising healthy sperm.

Track 12 – Stress relief (for both of you)

The tracks are all mp3 files and you can download them by visiting this page on my website:

http://loisfrancis.com/fertility-resources

You will need this password:- GPR385FYF

CHARTING FERTILITY

This guide is aimed at helping you to understand how charting your temperature can help you in your efforts to conceive.

In the pages that follow I'll explain how to take and record your temperature and most importantly how to interpret the results.

I usually suggest to my patients that they consider charting for around 3 months to get familiar with their unique cycle and fertility signals. The more aware you become of your fertile window, the easier it is to time intercourse to make the most of your chances of conceiving.

I only suggest charting for 3 months if your pattern is pretty stable from month to month. After that you can monitor your fertility by checking your cervical mucus, which can be done easily and discreetly when you visit the toilet.

Taking your temperature every morning at the same time sounds straightforward, but it does mean that it has to be your first waking thought each morning! It can set you up for the day focussing on your fertility, the best time to have sex, and take over normal life.

It can have a detrimental effect on your own and your partner's libido if making love becomes all about baby making and having sex "at the right time."

Having said that, I do think charting is useful to help you become more aware of your own fertile window. But there is so much more to getting pregnant than having sex at the right time. There is a lot you can do to improve your own and your partners fertility, reduce stress levels and enhance your overall health.

The chart can be downloaded from my website (use the same link as for the relaxations) and there lots of apps available now to help you record your temperature.

How to Chart Your Fertility

Fertility charting is all about getting familiar with your own cycle, identifying when you ovulate and your body's signals that tell you when you are about to ovulate. Charting will tell you if and when you have ovulated and you've passed your fertile window.

Although we're taught that the average menstrual cycle is 28 days and that we ovulate 14 days before the start of the next cycle, the length of cycle and timing of ovulation can vary by several days. It's really helpful to get an understanding of your body rhythms and cycles so that you can time intercourse to take place during your fertile window.

The lifespan of an egg is only 12 to 24 hours, it can even be as short as 6 hours. This may sound like an impossibly short time in which to have sex, but sperm can survive for up to 5 days waiting for the egg to be released! This means that you really have a window of opportunity in which you can aim to have sex daily if possible. The most likely days that intercourse will result in conception are the two days before ovulation and the day of ovulation.

Getting familiar with your fertility signals such as your cervical mucus can help you to focus your efforts more effectively. Couples who are aware of their fertile time and focus intercourse during this time have been found to have much higher conception rates than couples who are unaware of their most fertile time.

The primary fertility signs are:

- your basal body temperature (BBT) which rises after ovulation.
- your cervical fluid, sometimes called cervical mucus (CM) which gets increasingly wet, clear and stretchy as ovulation approaches.

The chart on the next page illustrates the following:

the cycle phases,

the hormones that are released through the cycle

the fertile window

typical temperature patterns

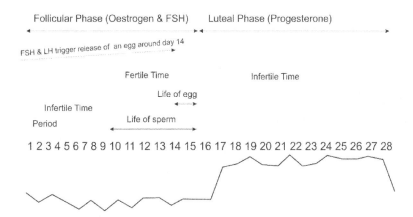

Charting your fertility signs helps you to find your optimum 3 day window, so that you can best time intercourse to get pregnant.

To maximize your conception chances, it is recommended to have intercourse every day or AT LEAST every other day during your fertile time until a clear and sustained thermal shift can be detected on your chart.

The chart on the next page shows how fertility charting can show you how to identify your fertile days and your ovulation date.

Temperature will often dip just before ovulation, and a sharp rise will show that ovulation has taken place. On this chart intercourse was timed to take place from days 11 through 14. As you can see, the temperature remained high indicating pregnancy.

174

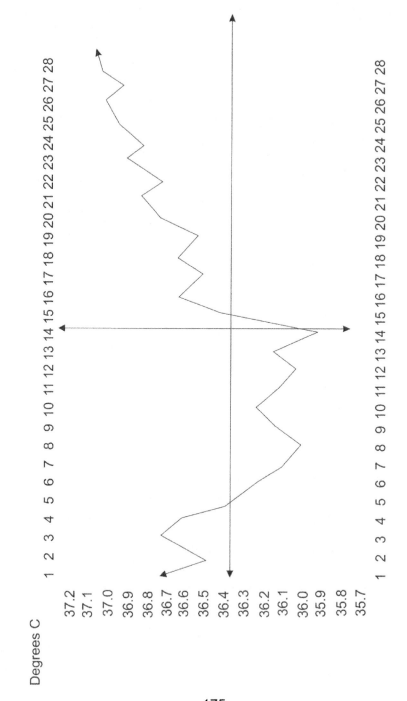

Noting & Recording Your Temperature

In order to get started you'll either need to print off the temperature chart from my website, or use one of the on-line services or an i-phone app.

You will also need a BBT thermometer or an accurate digital fever thermometer. Depending on your particular thermometer, you will record your temperature either in celsius or fahrenheit.

Your menstrual cycle and your fertility chart start on the first day of full menstrual bleeding ie full red flow, not spotting. This is day one of your cycle.

Your primary fertility signs are your basal body temperature (BBT) and cervical fluid or mucous. These are the signs that you need to record to get a reliable interpretation of when you are likely to ovulate.

Checking your primary fertility signs should only take a few minutes each day to observe and record your signs.

 The essential signs to check are:

your waking temperature

your cervical fluid observations

when you have menstrual bleeding

Your basal body temperature (BBT) should be measured when you wake up in the morning using an inexpensive special thermometer that you can buy at your drugstore or pharmacy.   Ask for a BBT or fertility thermometer.

In this section we'll focus on recording your temperature accurately so that you get useful, reliable information.

Some important guidelines to follow when taking your BBT

Your temperature data will be most reliable if you follow these guidelines. Not following these guidelines may make your chart difficult to read and may make detecting ovulation more difficult as well.

The closer you can get to the ideal the more accurate and reliable your ovulation detection, analysis and interpretation will be. Take your temperature before doing anything else including eating, drinking or going to the bathroom. If circumstances arise that prevent you from taking your temperature right away, take it as soon as you are able and make a note of the circumstances.

- Take your temperature before rising in the morning as any activity can raise your BBT.
- Take your temperature at the same time every morning.
- Take your temperature after at least three consecutive hours of sleep.

- Record your temperature on your chart soon after you take it since most thermometers only store a reading until the next use. You may want to keep your chart or a notepad on your bedside table.

Most women prefer to take their temperatures orally, however, when temperature patterns are unclear, switching to vaginal temperature-taking for the next cycle sometimes makes the pattern clearer. Always do one or the other ie don't take your temperature orally one day and vaginally the next.

If you use a heating pad or electric blanket, keep it at the same setting throughout your cycle. Make a note of its use.

FACTORS THAT CAN INFLUENCE YOUR BBT

There are certain factors that can influence your basal body temperature. These should be noted on your chart. These factors, should they apply to you, will usually not make charting and chart analysis impossible, especially if they occur only rarely, though it may be more challenging. In most cases, even when these factors apply on an ongoing basis, they will not skew your data so much that reading the chart is impossible.

The following factors may influence your BBT and should be noted in your chart data:

- Fever, cold, sore throat

- illness and infections (even those that do not produce a fever)
- drugs and medications
- alcohol
- smoking (if you smoke, you should consider quitting before you try to get pregnant)
- emotional or physical stress
- excitement
- sleep disturbances (insomnia, night-waking, upsetting dreams, poor sleep)
- change in waking time
- jet lag/travel
- change of climate
- use of electric blanket
- change of room temperature
- breastfeeding

After ovulation, the corpus luteum produces the heat-inducing hormone, progesterone. The principal reproductive function of progesterone in the luteal phase is to help prepare the lining of the uterus for the implantation of a fertilized ovum.

Progesterone, however, also causes the resting body temperature to rise after ovulation. Because progesterone is only secreted in high levels after ovulation, it is only possible to confirm that you have ovulated. Your temperature will not predict ovulation.

Before ovulation, during your follicular phase, basal temperatures are relatively low. After ovulation, your basal body temperature rises sufficiently that you can see the difference between your pre-ovulation and post-ovulation temperatures when they are plotted on a graph.

A fertility chart that shows ovulation detected by BBT will show lower temperatures before ovulation, a rise (thermal shift), and then higher temperatures after ovulation. Ovulation usually occurs on the last day of lower temperatures.

Your BBT corresponds to the heat-inducing hormone progesterone. This is the only sign that you can observe on your own that can confirm that ovulation actually happened. It is the changes in cervical secretions that tell you that ovulation may be approaching.

Because your temperature increases quite dramatically just after ovulation has taken place, it is the sign that will best help you to precisely pinpoint the day that ovulation occurred.

The rise in temperature is usually about 0.4 degrees Fahrenheit or 0.2 degrees Celsius, but the rise may be as slight as 0.2 degrees Fahrenheit or 0.1 degrees Celsius or even less in some cases. The actual temperatures are less important than noting a pattern showing two levels of temperatures.

If there is no pregnancy, your temperature will stay elevated for 10-16 days, until the corpus luteum regresses. As progesterone levels drop dramatically, you will get your period. Your temperature normally drops at this time as well, though it is not unusual to have erratic or high temperatures during your period.

While measuring your BBT can help to pinpoint or confirm ovulation, it is important to observe this sign in conjunction with other signs as well, particularly your cervical fluid. Observing multiple signs allows for cross-checking in the case that one sign is ambiguous or affected by other factors.

You may be wondering how taking your temperature can be of use, when you only get a significant shift after ovulation. By charting your temperature consistently you can use the BBT-confirmed ovulation date from previous cycles to predict the ovulation date of future cycles.

Charting your temperature along with observing your cervical fluid can give you great peace of mind. You can actually see that you timed intercourse well and can then stop wondering about your fertility status and your timing.

Observing and Recording Cervical Secretions

Your cervical fluid is the fluid that is produced by your cervix as ovulation is approaching. It is sometimes called cervical mucous or cervical secretions. You can see and feel it in or outside your vagina. Cervical fluid changes throughout your cycle depending on your fertility status.

You can easily observe your cervical fluid when you go to the bathroom and wipe yourself after using the toilet. Some women produce copious amounts of cervical fluids which are visible on a panty liner.

Cervical fluid is one of the best signs to tell you when you are most fertile before ovulation. When oestrogen levels are high and you are most fertile, cervical fluid is slippery, stretchy and resembles raw egg white. It is observable at the cervix or as it passes into the vagina

When you are trying to conceive, it is recommended that you have intercourse whenever you observe fertile quality cervical fluid. Cervical fluid has similar properties to semen and serves similar functions: to support, nourish and transport sperm.

In a typical menstrual cycle, cervical fluid starts out scant and dry just after menstruation, becoming sticky or pasty, then creamy before the more fertile, slippery and egg white fluid is observed when you are most fertile around ovulation. After ovulation, cervical fluid is again scant and dry.

Ovulation usually occurs around the last day that fertile quality cervical fluid is observed. This is often called the "peak" day, even though it may not be the day where the most fertile cervical fluid is observed.

The easiest and most effective way to monitor the presence and quantity of oestrogen in your bloodstream is to examine your cervical fluid as it changes during your menstrual cycle. Observing these changes offers a primary fertility sign that can tell you a great deal about what is going on with your fertility.

When you are not fertile, at the beginning of your cycle and after ovulation, cervical fluid is dry and scant or sticky and cannot be penetrated by sperm. At these non-fertile times, the vagina is quite acidic and is even hostile to sperm. Cervical fluid at this time forms a barrier that plugs the cervical canal and prevents bacteria from entering the uterus.

As the presence of oestrogen dramatically increases as ovulation approaches, this stimulates the production of large amounts of cervical fluid that is thin, stretchy, watery and alkaline- and receptive to sperm penetration. This most fertile fluid is best described as resembling raw egg white.

The main function of fertile cervical fluid in reproduction is similar to that of semen: as a medium for sperm nourishment and migration. Sperm survival and migration after intercourse is important because intercourse is rarely timed to exactly coincide with ovulation. Fertile cervical fluid contains "swimming lanes" which help the sperm in their journey toward the egg.   Once in your reproductive tract in fertile cervical fluid, the sperm can wait for the egg to be released.

Successful fertilization depends on the storage and constant release of sperm to the female upper reproductive tract at around ovulation time. When this kind of cervical fluid is present, sperm can be nourished and transported within your reproductive tract.   This is why it is important not to wait for ovulation, but to have intercourse as soon as you begin to notice fertile cervical fluid.

This "egg white" fertile fluid is usually observed in the most fertile days just before ovulation, drying up quickly after ovulation.

Cervical fluid observations tell when you are most likely to be fertile and offer an excellent way to time baby-making intercourse. To know for sure that you have actually ovulated and are no longer fertile, you will need to chart your temperature as well and observe a thermal shift (temperature rise) on your chart.

The prime advantage of the cervical fluid sign is its ability to answer the question "Am I now fertile?" which is at least as relevant as the question "When did I ovulate?" It is not necessarily the same question.

While your cervical fluid pattern may vary from cycle to cycle and it may vary from woman to woman, a typical cervical fluid pattern looks like this:

Immediately following menstruation there is usually a dry feeling in the vagina and there is little or no cervical fluid.

After a few days of dryness, there is normally a cervical fluid that is best described as "sticky" or "pasty" but not wet. While this kind of cervical fluid is not conducive to sperm survival these days may be considered as "possibly fertile" if found before ovulation.

Following these "sticky" days, most women generally notice a cervical fluid that is best described as "creamy". This fluid may be white, yellow or beige in color and has the look and feel of lotion or cream. At this point the vagina may feel wet and this indicates possible increased fertility.

The most fertile cervical fluid now follows. This most fertile fluid looks and feels like raw egg white. It is slippery and may be stretched several inches between your fingers. It is usually clear and may be very watery. The vagina feels wet and lubricated. These days are considered most fertile. This is the fluid that is the most friendly and receptive to sperm. It looks a lot like semen and, like semen, can act as a transport for sperm.

After ovulation, fertile fluid dries up very quickly and the vagina remains more or less dry until the next cycle. Some women may notice small amounts of fertile-looking fluid after ovulation as the corpus luteum produces small amounts of estrogen, but you are not at all fertile after ovulation has been confirmed.

By observing and recording these fertility signs, you can see when you are fertile on a graph. The information can be analyzed and interpreted and the feedback lets you see when you are approaching ovulation, when you have already ovulated, when you should expect your period or a positive pregnancy test, along with other insights that will help you get pregnant and learn about your unique fertility pattern.

To maximize your chances of conception, keep having intercourse until ovulation is confirmed by a clear and sustained thermal shift as intercourse closer to ovulation is much more likely to get you pregnant.

When cervical fluid is scant or absent, it is more important to try to time intercourse for as close to ovulation as possible, since sperm will not be able to survive as long while waiting for the egg to be released.

Don't be tempted to use a regular lubricant, saliva or even egg white if you find that intercourse is uncomfortable because you have little cervical fluid. Look for a specialised lubricant such as Pre-Seed which is designed to be sperm friendly.

Arousal fluid feels a lot like fertile cervical fluid but is secreted by your vagina, while cervical fluid is produced by your cervix. Both feel wet and slippery and both help to make intercourse more pleasurable and comfortable. Arousal fluid, unlike fertile cervical fluid, may be felt at any time during your cycle when you feel sexually stimulated. It may also be felt for up to several hours after any kind of sexually arousing activity.

If you are checking your cervical fluid before having intercourse when you are already aroused, it will usually feel slippery and it may be hard to tell the difference between the two kinds of fluids. Though the fluids feel similar, arousal fluid usually feels slightly more watery and will not usually stretch much. To avoid confusion, it is recommended to check your cervical fluid when you are not feeling particularly aroused.

How to check for cervical fluid externally

The most convenient way to check your cervical fluid is to make observations when you go to the bathroom. When you wipe, you can note what, if anything, you find on the bathroom tissue. This will soon become second nature and you will find yourself noticing your cervical fluid every time you go to the bathroom. You can also use your clean fingers to check for cervical fluid at any time. You may also notice some cervical fluid in your underwear.

Things to notice when checking your cervical fluid:

- Does the vagina feel wet or dry?
- Is there any fluid on the tissue?
- How does it look?
- What color is it?
- What consistency is it?
- How much is there?
- How does it feel when you touch it?
- Can you stretch it between your thumb and index finger?

If you have trouble finding cervical fluid, you may consider checking it internally. If you check your cervical fluid by internal observation, only the method for gathering the fluid is different. Otherwise, follow the same steps and observations as for external observation noted above.

To collect cervical fluid internally, follow these steps:

- Insert two fingers in your vagina until you can feel your cervix.
- One finger should be on each side of the cervix.
- Press gently against your cervix.
- Collect the fluid by moving your fingers to the opening of the cervix.
- Remove your fingers and pull them apart slowly.
- Make your observations as outlined for external fluid observation.

How to record your cervical fluid observations

No matter how you observe your cervical fluid (with your fingers, toilet tissue, in your underwear or internally if necessary) the way to record it will be the same.

Always record your most fertile type of cervical fluid, even if you noticed more than one type of cervical fluid in a given day or even if it is scant. This is so you will not miss a potentially fertile day and so that you have a consistent way of keeping track of your cervical fluid from cycle to cycle.

Not everyone experiences every type of cervical fluid. Just record the types you do get. You may also have some cervical fluid that does not seem to "fit" perfectly into any category. In this case, record it in the most fertile category that best seems to fit. For example, if you notice in a day that you have cervical fluid that seems to fit somewhere in between creamy and slippery, record it as slippery. Likewise, if you get both creamy and slippery fluid in the same day, record slippery on your chart.

Dry: Record your cervical fluid as "dry" if you have no cervical fluid present at all; if you notice no cervical fluid in your underwear; and if the outside of your vagina feels dry.

You can expect to see dry days both before ovulation after your period and after ovulation. Record "dry" if you are not able to gather or see any cervical fluid, even if your vagina feels slightly moist inside.

Sticky: Record your cervical fluid as "sticky" if it is glue-like, gummy, stiff or crumbly and if it breaks easily and quickly and if it is not easily stretched. It will probably be yellowish or white, but could also be cloudy/clear. You may or may not see some sticky cervical fluid before and after ovulation.

Creamy: Record your cervical fluid as "creamy" if it is like hand lotion, white or yellow or cloudy/clear, like milk or cream, mayonnaise or like a flour/water solution. It may stretch slightly but not very much and break easily.

Wet: Enter "wet" if your cervical fluid is clear and most resembles water. It may be stretchy also. This cervical fluid is considered fertile and this may be your most fertile cervical fluid or you may get it before you get slippery cervical fluid or you may not get this type of fluid at all.

Slippery: This is your most fertile cervical fluid. Record "slippery" if your cervical fluid looks at all like raw egg white, is stretchy and clear, or clear tinged with white, or even clear tinged with pink. It also resembles semen (and has a lot of the same physical properties to allow the sperm to travel and be nourished). You should be able to stretch it between your thumb and index finger.

Spotting: Record "spotting" when you have any pink or dark red/brown spots that leave a small mark on your underwear or panty liner or that you only see when you wipe. If it does not require a pad or tampon, record it as spotting rather than menses. You may see spotting before or after your period, around the time of ovulation or around the time of implantation if you conceive. Do not start a new chart until you have red flow.

INTERPRETING YOUR CHART

In an ideal world fertility signs would come in the order expected and indicate ovulation for the correct day. While this is not always the case, this is the most usual charting pattern.

The regular ovulation pattern has the following characteristics:

- cervical fluid becomes increasingly wet as ovulation draws nearer
- cervical fluid dries up quickly soon before or soon after the temperature rise
- a single patch of egg white cervical fluid is observed in the days just before ovulation
- a temperature shift, showing a marked increase in temperatures after ovulation
- temperature rises in a single abrupt shift that is sustained throughout the luteal phase
- OPK is positive 12-36 hours before the rise
- OPK is only positive in the one or two days before ovulation
- Fertility Monitor shows a High reading in the days leading up to ovulation and a Peak reading the day before the rise

When all signs indicate increased fertility for the same days prior to ovulation, and the ovulation date is clear, the detection of ovulation and the chart analysis can be quite certain.

The analysis and interpretation is more reliable when several signs can be correlated and cross-checked. It is, however, quite possible to detect ovulation and increased fertility under less than ideal charting circumstances. The more signs that "match" the more reliable the interpretation will be.

The ease with which a chart may be interpreted depends on the reliability and accuracy of the data entered and the clarity of the chart pattern. This is why being consistent with your temperature taking is so important. With each cycle charted, interpreting the fertility chart becomes increasingly easier.

An ideal chart pattern shows all your fertility signs lined up to suggest the same ovulation date. In this case, detecting ovulation is fairly straightforward: when cervical fluid has dried up and a thermal shift of three days or more has been observed (temperatures are higher than the previous several temperature points for at least three days), ovulation can be detected for the day before the temperature shifted.

Chart patterns are not always perfectly clear, however, so sometimes a bit of extra interpretation and flexibility is needed. If you are trying to conceive, it is recommended to keep on considering that you could be fertile if ovulation cannot be clearly determined on your chart. If there is any doubt at all that ovulation has already passed, keep on considering yourself fertile to increase your chances of conception.

Further Resources

www.fertilityfriend.com offer a good service which is free. You can also download apps from their site.

About the Author

As I've mentioned through the book I'm an acupuncturist with 20 years experience of treating couples with fertility problems. This book started life as a small booklet which I gave to my patients and as my knowledge has grown, so did the book.

I'm also a qualified NLP practitioner which gave me the tools for talking my patients into a deeply relaxed state and then using hypnotic suggestion to help them visualize. These guided relaxations are a standard part of my treatment and I tailor them according to where a women is in her fertility journey.

My patients have told me that these relaxation sessions are incredibly helpful. Most say that they feel far less stressed through their fertility treatment, so it's no surprise that success rates are higher than average.

I really enjoy treating my fertility patients, it gives me great joy when they come in and announce that they are pregnant. I usually work with them through the pregnancy and it has been known for me to get a text at midnight at the airport announcing the safe arrival of a baby!

I'm also passionate about supporting your health through nutrition which is why I wrote the recipe book

Eating to Get Pregnant. Used in conjunction with this book, I'm certain that you will find your health and fertility improve.

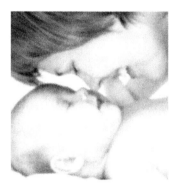

OTHER BOOKS BY LOIS FRANCIS

Eating to Get Pregnant

In this book you'll learn everything you need to know about eating to get pregnant. From balancing your blood sugar levels, detoxing, stocking your larder and fridge with fertility boosting foods to 100 carefully chosen recipes.

Brilliant Breakfasts
Luscious Lunches
Delicious Dinners
Tasty Treats

You'll never be short of ideas to create simple, nourishing, fertility boosting meals for yourself and your partner.

Available as a Kindle book or paperback only from Amazon.

Stop Stressing Start Living – the Complete Guide to Managing Stress and Creating the Life You Desire.

Overcome stress and lead a happy, healthy, stress-free life!

This book is for anyone who is suffering from stress and wants to turn their lives around. The book will enable you to:

1 Release your fears and anxiety.

2 Counteract the damage that negative stress has caused you.

3. Deal with the underlying cause(s) of your stress.

4. Feel inspired and motivated to create the life you really wish to experience.

Comes with audio version, guided relaxations which are downloaded from my website.

Available as a Kindle book or paperback only from Amazon.

A Perfect Human Being – a novel by Lois Francis

Lorna's life has been turned upside down.

She was in a job that she enjoyed but stuck in a comfort zone. She'd like to do more but lacked confidence in herself.

Her on/off boyfriend could be fun, but he lacked emotional maturity. The person she really admired would, in her view, never be interested in a relationship with her.

Her beloved Nan has died and the reading of the Will has unleashed a maelstrom of emotions and revealed family secrets she had been oblivious to.

In an effort to ingratiate himself with her, Lorna's boyfriend takes her out to a dodgy restaurant to celebrate her birthday. She ends up with food poisoning and acute appendicitis.

She wakes up in hospital after emergency surgery to see an angelic figure sitting on her bed. "You asked God for help, so here I am". Lorna is introduced to her guardian angels who are on a mission to help her re-evaluate her life and life purpose.

Lorna is introduced to three angels who drop in for conversations with her. Cheryl is a youthful, fun-loving angel who coaches her in using a simple tool to assess how well her life is working. David offers help with finances and Serena provides a sounding board for Lorna to explore new ideas.

With the support of her angels she learns how she can create the life she desires and help others to do the same. Old beliefs about what she can achieve are lovingly challenged and her energy and thoughts are channelled to be positive and creative.

By the end of the book you will find yourself rooting for Lorna, her friends and family, hoping that they will find the happiness that had eluded them.

If you are not currently in conversation with your own guardian angels, you will be pleased to know that the book introduces simple self-development ideas and techniques which you can apply to your own life, borrowing from the wisdom of Lorna's angels!

Available only from Amazon as a Kindle or paperback book.

The Relaxation Collection

The daily practise of relaxation and meditation has many positive benefits for your body, mind and feeling of well-being.

It switches off the stress response and helps to engage the "rest and digest" side of your autonomic nervous system. In turn, this optimises your digestion, lowers blood pressure and helps your body to eliminate toxins and renew worn out cells.

Studies show that people who take time out to relax and meditate on a regular basis respond better to stress, are calmer and more optimistic. They tend to have normal blood pressure and a lower risk of diabetes and heart problems.

Download my Relaxation Collection. The collection includes the following MP3 files: You receive all 8 tracks as a download package for just £17.

1. Enlightened communication
2. The Power Nap
3. Healing Light relaxation
4. Paradise relaxation
5. Relax into a deep sleep
6. River of Light relaxation
7. Seashore relaxation
8. Bonus track – Reclaim your Power.

Go to: http://loisfrancis.com/relaxations